"In this fascinating and quite unique book Devan Stahl and some of those who love her, offers a deep, rich and at points quite moving insight into what it means to live into enduring forms of illness. The interdisciplinary approach is powerful in the way that it allows us to see Devan's illness experiences from a variety of perspectives. . . .I commend this book and I pray that it both informs and changes people's views on what it means to live humanly in the company of enduring illness."

—JOHN SWINTON
Professor, School of Divinity, King's College University of Aberdeen

"In *Imaging and Imagining Illness*, Devan Stahl breaks new ground in the now well-populated field of illness writing. Combining personal memoir, artwork, rigorous analyses from bioethics and medical humanities, and philosophical reflection, it offers fresh interdisciplinary insights into the experience of illness and disability in a technologized medical world. More than anything else I have read, Stahl's book shows the reader how the person in illness interweaves multiple perspectives to give meaning to their experience."

—JACKIE LEACH SCULLY
Executive Director, Policy Ethics and Life Sciences Research Centre

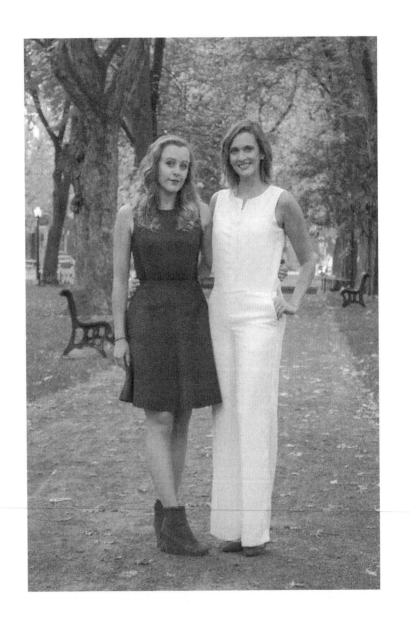

Imaging and Imagining Illness

Becoming Whole in a Broken Body

EDITED BY DEVAN STAHL

Foreword by
Rosemarie Garland-Thomson

CASCADE *Books* · Eugene, Oregon

IMAGING AND IMAGINING ILLNESS
Becoming Whole in a Broken Body

Cascade Books
An Imprint of Wipf and Stock Publishers
199 W. 8th Ave., Suite 3
Eugene, OR 97401

www.wipfandstock.com

PAPERBACK ISBN: 978-1-62564-837-2
HARDCOVER ISBN: 978-1-4982-8830-9
EBOOK ISBN: 987-1-5326-4029-2

Cataloguing-in-Publication data:

Names: Stahl, Devan | Goldin Stahl, Darian | Jones, Therese | Ostherr, Kirsten | Armour. Ellen T. | Bishop, Jeffrey P.

Title: Imaging and imagining illness : becoming whole in a broken body / edited by Devan Stahl

Description: Eugene, OR: Cascade Books, 2018 | Includes bibliographical references.

Identifiers: ISBN 978-1-62564-837-2 (paperback) | ISBN 978-1-4982-8830-9 (hardcover) | ISBN 987-1-5326-4029-2 (ebook)

Subjects: LCSH: Neuroimaging | Multiple Sclerosis | Human body—Religious aspects—Christianity | Diseases—Religious aspects—Christianity | Chronic Disease | Religion and Medicine | Technology Assessment, Biomedical | Nervous system—Diseases | Health—Religious aspects

Classification: R725.55 S713 2018 (paperback) | R725.55 (ebook)

Manufactured in the U.S.A.   01/19/18

Contents

Contributors

Devan Stahl, Assistant Professor of Clinical Ethics at the Center for Ethics and Humanities in the Life Sciences at Michigan State University.

Darian Goldin Stahl, PhD Student in the Centre for Interdisciplinary Studies in Society and Culture at Concordia University, Montreal. She is a Vanier Scholar who has been featured in dozens of solo and group exhibitions throughout the U.S. and Canada.

Therese Jones, Associate Professor, Center for Bioethics and Humanities at the University of Colorado Anschutz Medical Campus. She is the director of the Arts and Humanities in Healthcare Program; editor of the *Journal of Medical Humanities;* and lead editor of the *Health Humanities Reader.*

Kirsten Ostherr, Gladys Louise Fox Professor of English, Rice University, Houston, Texas. Her publications include *Cinematic Prophylaxis: Globalization and Contagion in the Discourse of World Health, Medical Visions: Producing the Patient through Film, Television, and Imaging Technologies, Science/Animation,* and *Applied Media Studies.*

Ellen T. Armour, E. Rhodes and Leona B. Carpenter Chair in Feminist Theology at Vanderbilt Divinity School. Director of the Carpenter Program in Religion, Gender, and Sexuality. Her most recent book is *Signs and Wonders: Theology After Modernity.*

Jeffrey P. Bishop, Professor of Philosophy and of Theological Studies, Tenet Endowed Chair in Health Care Ethics. Albert Gnaegi Center for Health Care Ethics. His recent book is *The Anticipatory Corpse: Medicine, Power, and the Care of the Dying.*

Foreword

Picturing Devan: From Clinical Specimen to Sacred Icon

ROSEMARIE GARLAND-THOMSON

Devan's story of transitioning from someone understood as well to someone understood as having multiple sclerosis is a story of coming to moral understanding. As Jackie Leach Scully explains in her 2008 book *Disability Bioethics: Moral Bodies, Moral Difference,* the experience of living as a person with chronic illness or disabilities can produce "experiential gestalts," or ways-of-knowing shaped by embodiment that are distinctive from the ways-of-knowing that nondisabled people's bodies develop as they interact with a world built to accommodate them. This "thinking through the variant body," as Scully calls it, can be a resource for moral understanding.

The moral understanding that emerges from Devan's story comes to us most explicitly through the reflective sections of this book written by Devan's sister Darian, Devan's teachers, and the scholars whose chapters follow Devan's own story. Therese Jones offers the anthropological concept of liminality to help explain the in-between-ness of illness and wellness. Kirsten Ostherr reflects on how technology pictures the previously unknowable. Ellen Armour ponders the increasingly wide chasm between divine authority and medical authority in our own self-understandings. Jeffrey Bishop considers a distinction between profane and sacred iconography. In this sense, the story and its elaborations move from secular to religious as the place of the divine occupies a more prominent position as this story progresses. Devan's story is intensely personal in tone and content, familiar to us who read illness memoirs. The explications of Devan's story make this feel more like a scholarly book than a personal narrative. What we have, then, is a hybrid of memoir and humanities scholarship. It is a unique, collective autopathography, which ultimately puts individual biography in the service of scholarly analysis.

My contribution to this book is to connect what Scully calls the "reconstructive narrative" at the heart of *Imaging and Imagining Illness* to a tradition of disability story making in the broadest sense that offers renewed ways of understanding and telling about the experience of living as a person with chronic illness or disability. In every case, this requires a translation of a patient story to a human story, from the clinical story to the lived story. In the case of Devan's story, it is a translation from a medical image to an aesthetic image, what eventually is revealed to be a translation from a profane to a sacred image. As Darian says, "The journey from patient to print is an act of many translations."[1]

In this retelling, Devan offers the MRIs and medical records to Darian, who translates them into the art that hangs on the office wall of Devan's mentor, Jeffrey Bishop. Darian's portrait of Devan is for Bishop an icon, a sacred object that incorporates—in the sense of embodying authentic corporeal being—the essence, reality, and perhaps even salvific properties of Devan. Bishop distinguishes Darian's artistic representation, which he understands as a sacred *icon*, from the profane representations of medicine, the *idols* of medical imagery that Darian transforms so that it imparts the authenticity and thus holiness of Devan. Devan's MRI and medical records are a form of idolatry, inauthentic representations of her because their authors do not recognize the holiness of her as God's rather than medicine's creation. Although Bishop does not

---

1. Goldin Stahl, "Lived Scans," 39, in this volume.

say all of this directly, the naming of Darian's art as icon confers sainthood on Devan, and secures her source of creation and purpose as a child of God. The representational trajectory from Devan as medical specimen—naked before the doctor, entombed in the MRI machine, curled like a fetus on the examining room floor—to Devan as icon beheld by the believer, Jeffrey Bishop, is the journey that this remarkable book recounts.

This is the account, then, of Devan's transition from MRI to icon, from medical specimen to sacred object. This translation in mode of representation, the book in its entirety suggests, is a salvation for Devan, a shift from a secular body to a holy body. Devan expresses that move in being as sharing her "scars" not her "wounds," suggesting the admirable restraint I appreciate in a story of suffering. Scars, of course, are our history, etched in the flesh, a remnant of our suffering. In telling our scars rather than wounds, we emphasize the resolution at the end of the story rather than the catastrophe that begins it. At the core of this collective story is recognition, legibility. Devan literally sees herself anew through Darian's images, transformed from a clinical image to a family picture. And the scholarly explications are testimonies of recognition of Devan transitioning from the state of temporary wellness into patient and on to at least survivor and at most sacred icon. Here and in other reconstructive narratives, there is a sense throughout of wisdom and wonder gained that comprise the narrative arc of living with illness and disability.

Imaging and Imagining Illness is in the tradition of re-narrations by disabled women writers. These are offerings, thoughtful and complex meditations about living with chronic illness and disability that imagine how we might accept if not even welcome such an inevitable entry into our lives. In one such offering, *The Rejected Body: Feminist Philosophical Reflections on Disability*, Susan Wendell concludes of her life with chronic illness, "I would joyfully accept a cure, but I do not need one."[2] Accepting disability as a legitimate human experience rather than an anomalous one

2. Wendell, *The Rejected Body: Feminist Philosophical Reflections on Disability*, 84.

transforms an experience understood as passive suffering and an identity engulfed by clinical narrative into a negotiation with the flesh that ultimately augments rather than reduces what might be considered her quality of life. In a more personal and writerly memoir, wonderfully titled *Waist High in the World: Life among the Nondisabled,* the wheelchair-using, Catholic, feminist writer Nancy Mairs offers a probing account of her own life with multiple sclerosis. Mairs's chronic illness and intensifying disabilities indeed have compromised the function of her body, but this way of being has also informed her sense of self. Both Wendell and Mairs directly address the primary temporal and narrative challenge of living with chronic illness and disability: that is, how to live fully as the now self without refusing that existence by reaching perpetually toward a lost then self or a cured future self.

Mairs echoes Wendell in that negotiation of ambiguity and open futures by telling us that if a cure were developed for MS she would take it, but that to flourish she does not need such a cure. Mairs offers no narrative here of chastening through suffering, but rather a deep understanding of the human condition and a sharp critique of social justice. Her utopian "task" in both writing the book and living her life, says Mairs, "is to conceptualize not merely a habitable body but a habitable world: a world that wants me in it."[3]

Darian's icons of being that transform Devan's MRIs preserve and honor the now self of chronic illness. The work, then, of Darian's representations here is to re-narrate, to tell another story to Devan about who she is. To use Mairs' words, the aesthetic representations present Devan with an image of a habitable body, one she can live in and live with, one that is not broken but beautiful, one fit to behold as a sacred object, what Jeffrey Bishop calls a "dark gift," not as a medical specimen. The translation of Devan's image from clinical to the sacred reaches as well toward making a habitable world, a world that wants the new self of Devan in it.

Aesthetic representations of chronic illness and disability conceptualize for us a world that wants disabled people, a world

---

3. Mairs, *Waist High in the World: Life among the Nondisabled,* 63.

that accommodates rather than eliminates the inherent human variations we think of as disabilities. Darian's translations of Devan's medical images contribute to the tradition of disabled artists re-narrating their own bodies through similar translations, what might more aptly be called incorporations. The disabled artists Katherine Sherwood and Laura Ferguson incorporate medical images of their bodies—for Sherwood, MRIs of her brain and for Ferguson, X-rays of her spine—into their self-portraits, transforming the medical images by incorporating them into their portraits. As the authors of their own bodies, of the visual stories they tell about their disabilities, these women recreate medical images as sacred images, as icons representing the bodies they inhabit, their own habitable bodies situated in a habitable world of their own creation.

A cerebral hemorrhage in 1997 transformed artist Katherine Sherwood's paintings by transforming her body. She changed from being a right-handed artist to a left-handed artist, a shift in technique and aesthetic production that led to a shift in content as she began to represent her own face with the image of her own medical portrait, her MRI.[4] She worked with larger canvasses, new implements, a different color palette, and a new body. In her series of self-portraits called "After Images," Sherwood re-narrates the 19th century tradition of the odalisque, the reclining nude woman offered up to the male gaze by artists such as Ingres, Lefebvre, Delacroix, Manet, and Matisse. By substituting the female face with her own MRI and adding her own leg braces and canes, Sherwood claims the tradition as her own with the costuming, if you will, of her own disability to transform and claim as her own Ingres' "Grande Odalisque" and "Reclining Nude" and Manet's "Olympia." These odalisques with disabilities insist on the womanly dignity and full humanity that the ways of being we think of as disabilities and illness are often imagined as rescinding.

4. Sherwood, "How a Cerebral Hemorrhage Altered My Art."

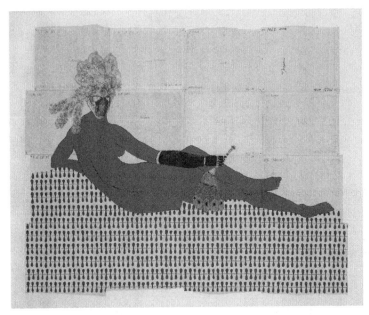

"After Ingres," Mixed media on found linen, 78" x 105," 2014[5]

The painter Laura Ferguson also incorporates contemporary medical imaging technologies that picture her "curving spine" in her self-portraits to create what she calls a "visual autobiography, telling the story of the life of my body." These portraits create a sense of flesh that is at once both opaque and transparent. "I draw myself from the inside out," Ferguson writes.[6] The conventions of painting bestow on her work a sense of sacred iconography, a feeling that the image is inhabited, that the flesh is animated. For Ferguson, this "conscious inhabiting of my body is at the core of my art." Like Darian's pictures of Devan, Ferguson's imagery, she tells us, takes "anatomy out of the realm of the medical and return[s] it to the personal."[7]

5. Courtesy of the Artist. All rights reserved. For more see http://katherinesherwood.com/.

6. Ferguson, "The Consciousness of the Body," http://www.lauraferguson .net/about-the-art/.

7. Ibid.

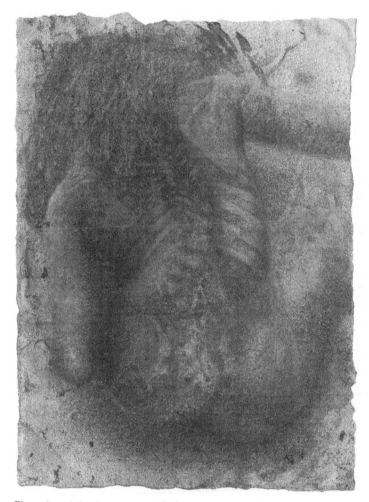

Figure imagining inner space, oils, bronze powder, charcoal, pastel, and oil crayon on paper, 14.5" x 11," 2004.[8]

Medical imaging technologies represent the matter beneath human flesh, endowing their images with an authoritative realism. This revelation of our interiority through MRIs and X-rays is taken to be medical truth, and thus incontrovertible truth. Its revelations

8. Courtesy of the Artist. All rights reserved. For more see http://www .lauraferguson.net/.

are assumed to display to the doctors our pathology, what's wrong with us and what demands correction. Because we have no direct visual access to our own interiority, these images have revelatory potential for us in literally witnessing our own internal being. Yet the narrow clinical use of these images for diagnostic or treatment purposes limits the potential of these pictures for self-knowledge and self-representation. We don't tend to understand these images as sacred revelations of our interiority because their utility is so circumscribed by the clinical setting in which they are produced and consumed. However, when these pictures of our deepest internal selves, some versions of our souls perhaps, move from the clinic to the work of art, we see ourselves pictured anew. This realism of our interiority takes on new resonance as it shifts from the medical to the aesthetic in our understanding of its representational work. So, the medical image becomes, as Jeffrey Bishop suggests, a sacred image of our interior, pictures of our brains or spines infused with aesthetic conventions that can suggest our essences, at the least, and our souls at most.

The self-portrait of disabled artist Riva Lehrer called "66 Degrees," alludes to this revelation of sacred interiority by directly representing the view of her own spine, shaped from birth by spina bifida.[9] The recognizable medical imaging that intentionally jars in Sherwood's portraits gives way in Lehrer's self-portrait to a kind of magical realism in which we see the artist's curved spine as an image emerged onto her skin, displayed for us in a pose as she would display herself to her medical visual interlocutors. But no longer in the clinic, rather in a swampy golden rain forest, festooned with a gilded robe worthy of a Byzantine saint or martyr, she bares the truth of her body as a sacred icon for us to witness. What Riva Lehrer's self-portrait adds most fully to the genre of disabled women's transformation of the medical into the aesthetic is the element of wonder. We have a sense in Lehrer's picture of witnessing a sacred image, of beholding a rewritten passion play in the restrained image of Lehrer in the primordial pool. Her pose and costuming at once allude to rewrite the sacred scenes of the baptism and the

9. Lehrer, *66 Degrees*, https://www.rivalehrerart.com/66degrees.

crucifixion. What we have in Lehrer's self-portrait is the intensely enfleshed woman displaying her spinal stigmata in an intimate act of sacred witnessing and revelation that renders her viewers pilgrims and their exchange holy.

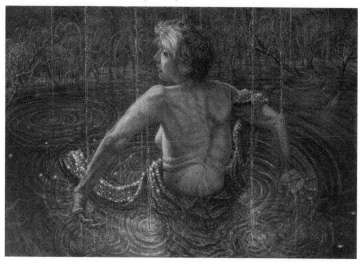

"66 Degrees," Acrylic on wood panel, 24" x 36," 2016[10]

All of these portraits of disability and chronic illness as sacred icons accrue the power of representing the truth of embodiment by invoking the ancient tradition of wonder at the heart of religious iconography. Medical iconography reduces with its aim of diagnosing and pathologizing. In contrast, aesthetic iconography enlivens, as the work of Darian's prints of Devan and the self-portraits of the disabled artists Sherwood, Ferguson, and particularly Lehrer amply show. These are images of flourishing rather than languishing. These are portraits of ensoulment rather than pictures of pathology. These images evoke wonder rather than distress. These narratives of being are part of a tradition to which *Imaging and Imagining Illness: Becoming Whole in a Broken Body* newly contributes. Collectively, the cultural work of these re-imaginings and re-narrations work toward strengthening the cultural,

10. Courtesy of the Artist. All rights reserved. For more see https://www.rivalehrerart.com.

Acknowledgments

When I was first diagnosed with multiple sclerosis, I could not have imagined all the amazing people my diagnosis would bring me into contact with and all the ways my world would be opened up. What initially seemed to be the worst news I ever received turned out to be the most transformative.

This book was several years in the making and I am grateful to all those who made it possible, including my collaborators, mentors, and fellow disability advocates, as well as the friends and family who endlessly encourage me. This project would not have been possible without her insights, skills, and compassion. I am proud to call her both my sister and my collaborator. Darian saw what I needed to be well even before I did, and for that, I will be forever grateful. Our collaboration has made my scholarly work more meaningful and my personal life richer. Darian continues to challenge and inspire me through her art and I have been fortunate to see her art affect many others as well. She is an incredible artist, as I am sure will be obvious to all those who see her art for the first time in this volume.

I am grateful that my Ph.D. advisor, Jeffrey P. Bishop, encouraged me to broaden my initial ideas into this edited volume. Then and now, Dr. Bishop has helped me to think bigger and aim higher. Much of my success is a result of his excellent mentorship and guidance. Additional thanks to the other scholars who agreed to write chapters for this work: Therese Jones, Kirsten Ostherr, Ellen Armour, and Rosemarie Garland-Thomson. Thank you for all of your encouragement and your enthusiastic agreement to support this project. Thanks also to the artists Riva Lehrer, Katherine Sherwood, and Laura Ferguson, for agreeing to have their art featured in this book. Your art has been an inspiration to myself, Darian, and so many others.

I am also thankful for the supportive colleagues and friends in my life. In particular, my Vanderbilt squad, Drs. Carolyn J Davis, Jennifer Adler, Lydia Willsky-Ciollo, and Leah Payne for being my support network. My Saint Louis University cohort, including Rachelle Barina and Emily Trancik who were my companions in doctoral work. And of course, to my loving husband, Christopher Bruce Wright, who supports me in my academic and advocacy endeavors and spent many nights reading drafts of this manuscript.

I would like to thank all those who listened to early drafts and presentations of this book, including the participants of the 2014 International Health Humanities Conference, who eagerly encouraged Darian and I to continue with our collaboration, as well as the Religion and Disabilities Studies Unit of the American Academy of Religion and the American Society for Bioethics and Humanities.

Finally, I am thankful to Nancy Mairs, Kay Toombs, Jackie Leach Scully and all the other authors who inspired me to write myself into well-being.

Introduction

For the past ten years, I have lived with multiple sclerosis (MS). MS has changed the way my body functions, how I experience and live in the world, and how I understand myself. Through most of my illness journey, I have appeared able-bodied. My outward body masks the lesions present in my brain, which can cause me to lose sensation in my limbs, my vision, and my memory. Sharing my illness story—my pathography—requires a certain amount of vulnerability. Vulnerability is nothing to be romanticized; it is difficult and often dangerous. Many people with chronic illnesses or other hidden disabilities never share their stories, for fear they will be pitied, marginalized, or preyed upon. Sharing illness stories is risky. Yet, sharing our vulnerabilities can also be cathartic, empowering, and community building. In this volume, I share a portion of my ever-growing pathography with a group of scholars doing interdisciplinary work on the body. They interpret and build upon my story, offering their unique insights on the place of the body in medicine and the wider culture.

THE CLINICAL VIEW AND THE LIVED EXPERIENCE

Multiple sclerosis is a chronic and disabling neurological disease, which affects the conduction of nerve impulses and the integrity of nerve signals in the central nervous system (most typically the brain stem and spinal cord white matter).[11] MS is an autoimmune disease, which means a person's immune system attacks the nervous system and, in the case of MS, destroys myelin, the insulating material that forms a sheath around neurons. As a demyelinating disease, MS affects the ability of nerve cells in the brain and spinal cord to communicate with each other effectively, creating lesions in the brain and spine.[12] Scientists do not know what causes MS, but as a twenty-something-year-old white woman of Northern European decent, I fit the profile of persons most likely to be diagnosed with MS.[13]

The clinical picture of MS says very little about how I live with or experience MS. I do not directly experience the scars on my brain, even though MRI scans have allowed me to see them. I experience fatigue and relapsing symptoms that cause my feet, legs, and eyes to work differently. Knowing my diagnosis, however, I am constantly aware of my MS. Every trip, every fumble, every bleary-eyed morning and tired afternoon is now replete with deeper meanings. Discerning "normal" bodily limitations from impending relapse is no easy task. MS affects how I interact with the world and how I interpret the meaning of my body and its coherency with my identity and self-perception.

Becoming ill can be a fragmenting and isolating experience. Medicine rarely offers the kind of consolation or soul-care that patients need when confronted with chronic illness. Over the past ten years or so, I have encountered deeply caring and thoughtful physicians (and even more nurses) as well as callous and thoughtless ones. Medical technology is not responsible for some physicians' tendency to objectify the body, but because my disease is most easily visible through MRI scans, many of my physicians have tended to spend more time looking at my scans than looking at me in our clinical encounters.

---

11. Traugott, "Evidence for Immunopathogenesis," in Cook (ed.), *Handbook of Multiple Sclerosis*, 163–86.

12. Wu and Alvarez, "The Immunopathophysiology of Multiple Sclerosis," 257–78.

13. Wingerchuk et al. *Multiple Sclerosis*, 263–81.

I fear that advanced medical imaging technologies may exacerbate the tendency to see patients primarily through their represented images. Certainly, the invention of sophisticated medical imaging technologies has made diagnosis much more efficient and has undoubtedly saved lives. I am grateful that my first neurologist had access to my MRI scans so that I did not need additional testing before I was finally diagnosed with MS. As efficient as the MRI machine is and as good as my physician was at diagnosing my disease, however, my MRI scans limit me. These scans present a single, albeit necessary picture of MS. My MRI scans obscure as much as they reveal. How I experience illness is shaped by my encounters with my family, community, professional colleagues, culture, and environment. Medicine alone cannot account for my experience of MS, which is why I have reached beyond the field of biomedicine to help inform how I understand my disease.

READING AND WRITING MS

When I was diagnosed with MS, I knew little about the disease. It took time for me to be able to tell people about my diagnosis. I encountered other MS patients first through narrative. Nancy Mairs was my first illness companion. Mairs' bold honesty about her triumphs and hardships living with MS helped me to imagine my future with the same humor and grace.[14] I was never able to meet Mairs before she died in 2016, but I will be forever grateful that she had the courage to write about her life with MS. Through Mairs' narrative honesty, I became convinced that part of my healing would come through writing my own narrative. Writing became a way for me to access my feelings, my evolving interpretation of my body, and my reemerging identity.

Most illness narratives are triumphant—the narrator overcomes a terrible illness, only to be reshaped by the experience. MS is chronic and without a cure, so there is little chance that my own narrative will be one of triumph. Instead, my narrative is one of

14. Mairs, *Waist-High in the World.*

living with and coming to terms with a progressive and disabling illness. Narrative writing has been one habit I have taken up that has helped me to reflect upon how illness shapes my life. Speaking illness is difficult. Writing, however, allows for critical distance. In writing about my illness, I did not have to get the words right the first time. I could catalogue and reflect on how MS disrupted what I believed to be the shape and purpose of my embodied life.

My emerging illness identity was not something I was able to share with my physicians. S. Kay Toombs, a phenomenologist with MS, helped me to understand why I felt so uncomfortable in the medical arena. By explaining how patients and doctors interpret illness differently, I was able to understand what I found so discomforting about how my doctors spoke about my illness and interacted with my body.[15] Whereas physicians learn about a thing called "MS" and how to see it in an MRI scan, I cannot separate MS from my *experience* of MS. I do not experience my illness as a bright spot in my brain, as it is represented through an MRI scan. Physicians need to break the body up, to see its parts in order to understand what is causing its dysfunction. I experience MS, on the other hand, as an array of spontaneous symptoms that affect my lived experience. Medicine demands objective data, patients have subjective experiences. The urge to bridge the disconnect that can occur between doctors and patients is part of the reason I ended up as a bioethicist.

The courage of women such as Mairs and Toombs inspired me to write my narrative and explore my illness through disciplines outside of medicine. Sharing my pathography with others, however, took time. Pastor Nadia Bolz-Weber advises public speakers to share their scars and not their wounds.[16] To tell a compelling story, you need to ensure you do not bleed all over your audience. If the point is to share a lesson, something you have learned from your experience, you do not want your audience to feel they need to comfort you or clean up your mess. To teach through experience, you must be vulnerable, but you must also be confident. To

15. Toombs, *The Meaning of Illness.*
16. Bolz-Weber, "Seeing the Underside and Seeing God."

share the stories of your life with illness—your pathography—as I hope to do, requires a degree of reconciliation and self-acceptance. My journey in illness will last a lifetime, but I learned to accept illness as a part of myself—a part of my embodied experience, which shapes who I am and how I see and interact with the world. The journey of self-acceptance requires time and reflection, but is never complete. The relapsing and remitting nature of my disease means that I can never predict how it will affect me. I cannot know what is to come or how well I will cope, but I do have faith that ultimately all will be well. Through telling my story, I share my scars, and while I hope they do not bleed, I do want them to unsettle and provoke.

OPENING UP THE FIELD OF INTERPRETATION

To get the medical care that I need to manage my MS symptoms, I subject myself to the medical gaze. I willingly concede control of my body to my physicians, trusting they have the expertise needed to monitor my disease, prescribe medication, and interpret my symptoms. I do not have to agree with my physicians' assessments, but I do need to grant them some authority over my body if I want to gain access to their expertise and treatments. Relinquishing interpretative and bodily control can be difficult, however, particularly when medical categories do not always capture my evolving understanding of my illness. I am not satisfied to grant medicine sole interpretation of my body. Medicine's interpretative power is culturally formidable, but the field of medical science is not singular in its attention to the human body. Artists, philosophers, theologians, anthropologists, bioethicists, and many other scholars write out of rich traditions seeking to interpret the meaning of embodiment and illness.

The idea for this volume began when I shared my MRI scans with my sister, Darian Goldin Stahl. Darian is a print artist who now uses my scans in her artwork. Viewing Darian's art, I learn new things about myself that would have remained inaccessible without allowing her to interpret my body through her discipline. Our collaboration has shaped the way I understand my life with illness and it has shaped how she understands the purpose of her art. We have been mutually enriched by this collaboration.

The beauty and meaning created from sharing my story and my images with Darian inspired me to open our collaboration to others. I want to take seriously the idea that bodies are socially constructed and that our cultural discourse shapes the values and meanings of that construction. Reading my narrative and looking at the same set of MRI scans, I believe different interpreters from different fields of inquiry will see different things and add to the discourse of the body. Acknowledging that all bodies contain an inherent irreducibility, I have asked other scholars to situate medical scans into their own field of inquiry. They will consider what importance or weight ought to be given to such images in our vision of the human person. What sort of "truth" are the images able to provide? How can these images be universalized or particularized? Can such a reductive image ever find coherence within one's body image? How can we understand such images alongside the "lived" body? Given the same narrative and set of medical images, my hope is that these scholars will offer unique contributions to the body's interpretation.

I begin this volume with a short pathography describing some of my interactions with the medical community and my initial diagnosis. I explain how I experience the process of MRI scans, interacting with clinicians, and the influence my illness has on my self-identity. Next, Darian Goldin Stahl supplies her interpretation of my illness and body image through her artist prints and accompanying descriptions. She adds her own remembrance of my diagnosis and how it affected her life and artistic career. Dr. Therese Jones then reflects upon my story and Darian's art through the lens of the medical humanities. Dr. Jones picks up the themes of liminality, pathography, and identity formation in illness. Dr. Kirsten Ostherr's chapter details the history of medical "technovision" and the ways in which patients can use creative forms of expression to reclaim their bodies. Using the lens of visual culture and media studies, Dr. Ostherr describes how patients can disrupt the biomedicalization of life and empower themselves in the digital age.

The final two chapters reflect on all four of the previous chapters, adding additional layers of meaning and interpretation. Dr. Ellen T. Armour writes as a theologian interested in biopower and resistance. Dr. Armour's chapter is concerned with how certain images and narratives can mirror or resist our modern ways of knowing and being in the world. Dr. Jeffrey P. Bishop, a physician and philosopher in bioethics, considers the power ontology of medicine, as well as patient empowerment and the dark gift of bodily frailty. Dr. Bishop emphasizes what is gained in self-giving.

I selected these contributors for their disciplinary expertise, but also because each author works across multiple disciplines in his or her engagement with medicine and the body. These authors are used to thinking about a single subject through multiple lenses, which will be evident in their contributions. Refusing to speak through a single lens, each opens up the possibilities for interpreting and situating the ill body. I end the volume by reflecting on what new insights I have gained through their writing. Bodies will always exceed the sum of their parts, and by expanding the interpretative lens of an individual body, I hope to point toward the body's complex and excessive nature.

BIBLIOGRAPHY

Bolz-Weber, Nadia. "Seeing the Underside and Seeing God: Tattoos, Tradition, and Grace." *On Being*. Podcast audio, October 23, 2014. https://onbeing. org/programs/nadia-bolz-weber-seeing-the-underside-and-seeing-god-tattoos-tradition-and-grace.

Cook, Stuart D. *Handbook of Multiple Sclerosis*. 3rd ed. New York: Taylor & Francis, 2005.

Mairs, Nancy. *Waist-High in the World: A Life among the Nondisabled*. Boston: Beacon, 1996.

Toombs, S. Kay. *The Meaning of Illness: A Phenomenological Account of the Different Perspectives of Physician and Patient*. Dordrecht, Netherlands: Kluwer Academic, 1993.

Wingerchuk, Dean M., Claudia F. Lucchinnetti, and John H. Noseworthy. "Multiple Sclerosis: Current Pathophysiological Concepts." *Laboratory Investigation* 81 (2001) 263–81.

Wu, Gregory F., and Enrique Alvarez. "The Immunopathophysiology of Multiple Sclerosis." *Neurologic Clinics* 29 (2011) 257–78.

I

Living into My Image

DEVAN STAHL

LIVING IN TIGHT SPACES

Pressure builds inside my chest as if it is being pushed from both the front and back. My breathing is shallow and restricted and I force myself to take long, deep breaths. A sensation of restlessness begins in my chest and slowly moves out to every inch of my body. Suddenly I feel like I am vibrating, as if at any moment my whole body is going to rip apart. I want to move, I have to move. Not moving requires holding back all the forces in my body that are desperately pushing outward. If this does not end soon I am going to break. Tears well up in my eyes, but I desperately try not to open them. Small streams run down my face and make my skin itch. Normally I would open my eyes and fan them, but I resist. I squeeze my eyelids tighter to drain the fluid. I know I shouldn't, but I open my eyes in an act of defiance. Now I see what I was dreading: the dark narrow walls of the tunnel just inches from my face. My eyes begin to cross as they try to focus on the crossbar attached to my head restraint. I quickly close my eyes again.

I never knew I had claustrophobia until I began receiving regular MRI exams. It takes all of my will power not to yank out my IV and scramble out of the machine. Of course, I agreed to be in that scanner; I agreed it was best for my health to subject myself to the scan and I know that if I stop in the middle, I will be forced to start the whole process over again. I am a willing participant in this uncomfortable process because it is necessary for my "medical treatment plan" and my doctor ordered it. I am chronically ill and I require constant monitoring. I have never asked to be sedated, partly out of cowardice and partly out of arrogance. I do not like asking for drugs. I should learn to conquer this feeling. I should learn to be more meditative. Perhaps I can turn this fear into an opportunity for contemplative spiritual practice. No luck so far with that particular ambition.

The whole MRI production begins at the hospital, a fine place to be if you work there, but a dreadful one if you are ill. After filling out my preliminary intake forms, I am asked to undress and put on a hospital gown, two if the gown is flimsy. Better safe than sorry. I have found the standards for the clothes I can wear during the exam vary depending on the lab. I once had a rather awkward conversation with a radiology technician about my bra. He was an older, slightly grizzly looking man who introduced himself by asking where I bought my bra. In my vulnerable position, I did not immediately ask why he wanted to know. I assumed he was a professional with a point. Apparently, Victoria Secret bras use a plastic underwire, which is perfectly fine in the MRI scanner. Regardless, he informed me, a metal underwire, like the metal zipper and button on my jeans, would vibrate during the exam, "which some women rather enjoy." This comment left me in the rather awkward position of having to decide whether I should leave my clothes on and allow this man to think I was "enjoying" the exam, or take them off and feel cold for the next two hours. My advice: leave your clothes on if you can. Hospitals are cold and the inside of an MRI scanner is no different. Do not allow perverted old men to convince you not to take your clothes off, as counterintuitive as that may sound. It never ceases to amaze me what some men think is appropriate to say to a young female patient.

After I change, I sit on a locker-room bench, waiting for a technician to prepare the machine, finish with the previous patient, or tell jokes about my undergarments. I can only guess what they are doing behind those doors. When I finally enter the lab, a tech fits me with an IV so he can later inject me with contrast dye. I have very small veins and when I go for blood draws, nurses often require several attempts to strike just the right place. The nurses who know me give me a heating pack and use infant needles. Radiology technicians have no such sensitivities and I have been known to faint or become nauseous after an IV insertion. I am not afraid of needles, so the immediate physical reaction I sometimes have to an IV is frustrating and somewhat embarrassing. One prick of that large needle and the room begins to spin. Thankfully, I have never vomited on a tech and I pride myself on this feat.

When I lie down on the scanner, the tech secures my head into place so I cannot move it. It is terribly uncomfortable and my neck is usually sore after the exam. Someone hands me a buzzer in case I need to speak with the techs, which I have never used, and earplugs to drown out the noise of the machine. There is no drowning out the noise of the loud machine, and worse still, the noise it produces is completely arrhythmic. There is simply no chance of making a song or jingle out of the pulsing, erratic sounds. I have tried. There is no sensation I can escape into during the process. I try to avoid seeing, hearing, touching or even smelling anything in the narrow walls of the scanner. The best I can do is escape into my own thoughts, but given the reason for having the scan in the first place, my thoughts can quickly turn anxious. The whole process can take over two hours and still longer if I move to adjust my aching body. The result of my efforts is hundreds of computer-generated images of my body, from my lower spine to the top of my head.

LIVING IN NUMBNESS

I vividly remember the first time I ever laid eyes upon my MR images. I was twenty-two and had just finished my first semester of divinity school in the buckle of the Bible Belt. I had left my conservative denomination for one that allowed female clergy and I was feeling empowered. I was even beginning to reconsider ordination, a dream I had abandoned at the age of fourteen when my minister told me that, while I was very bright, God did not call women to leadership in the church. Perhaps God wanted me to *marry* a minister and I was getting my wires crossed. Then and now, I find all the "calling" metaphors in church-talk confusing; I have never heard God's voice directly. Embarrassed to admit this fact, as I believed it revealed a lack of faith on my part, I agreed my pastor must be right. Only after studying religion in college did I learn that many Christian denominations ordain women and they managed to do so reading the same Bible and without crossing out a single line of Scripture.

I chose to go to Vanderbilt Divinity School because of its progressive reputation. I soon acquired a group of diverse friends with a variety of opinions and belief systems. I was having a blast. Contrary to popular opinion, the South is full of open-minded people and seminarians can be some of the most socially progressive people you will ever meet. My colleagues were passionate, energetic, and they wanted to change the world. We rallied for marriage equality one week and held Southern-style revivals the next.

Then my feet went numb and the fun stopped. A sort of tingling sensation began at my feet and started to creep up my legs slowly. It almost felt as if my feet were asleep, but the tingling lasted for days. Although the lack of sensation I experienced allowed me to wear my highest heels without discomfort, I figured I should probably go to a doctor. At twenty-two I was naïve, but not grossly irresponsible. After attempting to make a hospital appointment only to be told I would have to wait eight weeks to see a doctor, I drove myself to a walk-in clinic. Unsurprisingly, the physicians there had no idea what was wrong with me. The sensation slowly dissipated and within a few weeks had completely vanished. I spent the following months seeing a variety of physicians who all had their own tests to perform. The process was annoying and expensive, but I anticipated coming out of it just fine. I was a healthy, if somewhat clumsy, twenty-two-year-old, and I never expected anything was seriously wrong with me. More than anything, I was annoyed at the constant traveling, waiting times, and mundane questions the physicians asked.

Three months later I was given my first MRI scan and referred to a neurologist. It took the neurologist all of thirty seconds to diagnose me after examining my scans.

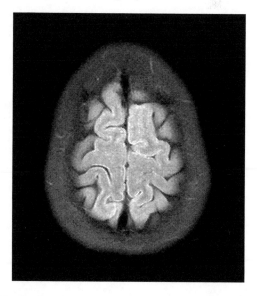

"It's MS!" he declared. I was speechless. MS? I did not see this coming. My mind raced.

How could he tell? What is he seeing? What is going to happen to me? Didn't I see this coming? Didn't I do an Internet search on this? Didn't the other doctors tell me I was going to be all right? Were they lying? Did they know? Did they suspect? How can he know I have a devastating illness just looking at those gray blobs? What is MS? It's bad . . . it's neurological . . . it's debilitating . . . wait,

I know someone with MS . . . a woman who goes to my church has MS. Every Sunday she comes and goes in a van because she is a quadriplegic.

A lump begins to form in my throat. I know this feeling. I hate this feeling. I know what is coming and I know I cannot stop it. I used to hate crying in front of other people (now I only exceedingly dislike it). I was trying to cultivate the habits of a strong female leader and at twenty-two crying made me feel powerless and pathetic. My rather insensitive physician pushed a box of tissues my way without taking his eyes off the computer screen containing my MRI scans. I tried to pull myself together.

"How can you be sure?" I managed. He looked confused. "I'm not sure what you are seeing in those pictures," I followed up.

"I'm a specialist" he assured me, in his most proud and patronizing tone. "I know what I am looking for."

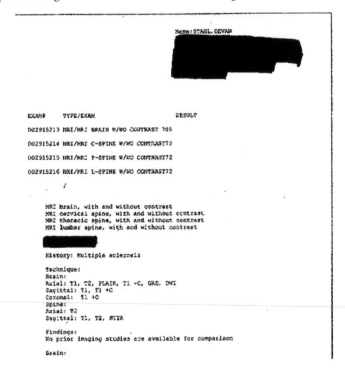

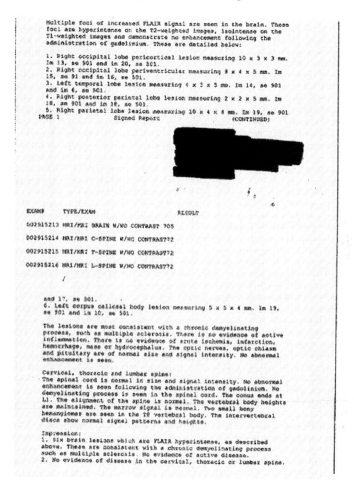

Multiple foci of increased FLAIR signal are seen in the brain. These foci are hyperintense on the T2-weighted images, isointense on the T1-weighted images and demonstrate no enhancement following the administration of gadolinium. These are detailed below:

1. Right occipital lobe pericortical lesion measuring 10 x 3 x 3 mm. Im 13, se 901 and im 20, se 801.
2. Right occipital lobe periventricular measuring 8 x 4 x 5 mm. Im 15, se 91 and im 16, se 101.
3. Left temporal lobe lesion measuring 4 x 3 x 5 mm. Im 14, se 901 and im 6, se 801.
4. Right posterior parietal lobe lesion measuring 2 x 2 x 5 mm. Im 18, se 901 and im 18, se 501.
5. Right parietal lobe lesion measuring 10 x 4 x 4 mm. Im 19, se 901

PAGE 1   Signed Report   (CONTINUED)

EXAM#   TYPE/EXAM   RESULT

002915213 MRI/MRI BRAIN W/WO CONTRAST 705

002915214 MRI/MRI C-SPINE W/WO CONTRAST?2

002915215 MRI/MRI T-SPINE W/WO CONTRAST?2

002915216 MRI/MRI L-SPINE W/WO CONTRAST?2

and 17, se 301.
6. Left corpus callosal body lesion measuring 5 x 5 x 4 mm. Im 19, se 901 and im 10, se 501.

The lesions are most consistent with a chronic demyelinating process, such as multiple sclerosis. There is no evidence of active inflammation. There is no evidence of acute ischemia, infarction, hemorrhage, mass or hydrocephalus. The optic nerves, optic chiasm and pituitary are of normal size and signal intensity. No abnormal enhancement is seen.

Cervical, thoracic and lumbar spine:
The spinal cord is normal in size and signal intensity. No abnormal enhancement is seen following the administration of gadolinium. No demyelinating process is seen in the spinal cord. The conus ends at L1. The alignment of the spine is normal. The vertebral body heights are maintained. The marrow signal is normal. Two small bony hemangiomas are seen in the T8 vertebral body. The intervertebral discs show normal signal patterns and heights.

Impression:
1. Six brain lesions which are FLAIR hyperintense, as described above. These are consistent with a chronic demyelinating process such as multiple sclerosis. No evidence of active disease.
2. No evidence of disease in the cervical, thoracic or lumbar spine.

My body shrinks in and I stare at the floor, then back at the computer, then back at the floor. All the energy leaves my body. I have no more questions. I am empty. I curl up in the fetal position and a large needle is inserted into my spine; my diagnosis is confirmed. I have multiple sclerosis.

The significance of this event took days to settle in. I was finally beginning to accept and appreciate my womanhood—including my female body—and what it might mean to be a strong feminist, and the diagnosis felt like a setback. Illness and disability would surely make me weak and make my goals in life, already lofty, harder to achieve than ever. What if I could not walk? What if I went blind? What if I lost my memory and could not be a scholar? And though my young feminist self was loath to admit it, I could not help but think, "Will anyone ever want to marry me or have children with me?"

I was unsure how to talk about the diagnosis; I had no voice for it yet, so instead I read. I read stories and memoirs from women living with MS, and I read theologies of disability to learn how others reconciled their faith with their present embodiment. After some time I began to out myself to my friends and family. I wanted support, but I dreaded being pitied, which seemed inevitable. To this day, I still struggle with who to tell about my illness and when. I do not bear any of the overt, physical signs of illness and so it is easy to avoid the subject. My illness has become a large part of my identity, however, and I cannot hide it away. People always expect you to be sad or strong about illness. They want you to fight it and keep it distant from yourself. People want you to persevere through it to give them hope. Others want you to be quiet about it and endure it like a dignified woman who would not dare to burden others with her troubles. In the past, I have felt repulsed by women who flaunt their illness and use it as a constant excuse. I am less sure now if there is a right or wrong way to live with a chronic illness. For me, constantly battling or pitying my own body feels like an exhausting snare of self-loathing.

LIVING AS A GUINEA PIG

Soon after my diagnosis, my neurologist asked if I wanted to enter a clinical trial he was conducting for a new MS medication. The offer was tempting; I feared I would be unable to afford the medical care I thought I would need. Already by this time, I was receiving medical bills I could not pay and was forced to ask my parents for financial help. Although I had a generous scholarship and a part-time job, it did not take long to go through all of my funds. I had very few options; I was totally broke and reluctant to ask my parents for more money. In an attempt to pay the bills I had already accumulated, I went to our university registrar to ask if there was any way the school could loan me money. Well, that is what I intended to ask for anyway. What came out of my mouth was an unsettling period of silence, followed by a protracted period of crying, interspersed with what I imagine were incomprehensible words of explanation. The poor man. Unsure of what I was trying to convey he asked if I needed to consult the school's counseling services. At no point in my preparation of the request did I imagine I would fall into a sniveling mess. When forced to explain the diagnosis, I lost all my nerve.

Thankfully, the school was able to help me with my bills, but after only a few months I had also used up all of my university health insurance and the drugs that my physician recommended would have cost me thousands of dollars a month. A clinical trial appeared to be my only real option. The trial offered me three distinct benefits: I would receive free medication, with a 2/3 chance of it *not* being a placebo (a probability my mother was none too happy about); the drug was taken orally rather than through injection; and I would be seen by a different neurologist so there would be no conflict of interest for my current doctor, who had proven himself to be incredibly insensitive time and time again. If he would rather be my scientist than my doctor, I was happy to let my neurologist change roles. My new neurologist was far kinder; his only major fault was that he continually asked me if I had gotten taller since our last visit. I have been 5'8 since I was thirteen, so the question always seemed bizarre and a bit infantilizing. Had he forgotten to check my age on the chart, or did he simply never learn how the growth process works? Perhaps my height never ceased to amaze him and this was the most polite expression he could muster in the presence of such a tall female figure. Maybe he thought it was a compliment, the physician's equivalent to "have you lost weight?"

Due to the drug's minor side effects, including macular edema and sudden heart failure (which I never told my mother about), the trial consisted of constant monitoring. I am convinced that only unemployed or graduate student patients could have possibly made time for all the appointments the trial required. Over

9

the course of four years, I had numerous MRIs, echocardiograms, electrocardiograms, pulmonary function tests, eye exams, blood tests, walking tests, dexterity tests, and memory tests (cruel, cruel tests that involved quickly solving math problems in my head). I became a clinic regular. I was well known to nurses and desk clerk, but it took me almost a year to begin to ask my now plethora of doctors and technicians questions concerning why I needed these tests and what the results indicated. "Does that seem normal?" became my constant refrain. Unfortunately, most of my exams were performed by techs that either could not or would not interpret my results in any sort of detail. As someone unfamiliar with the medical system, it took me a while to realize that none of the exams or tests I underwent was for my benefit. I was not receiving medical care; I was a guinea pig. I was testing a product. (I have subsequently learned many human research subjects mistakenly believe research is intended to offer them therapeutic benefit.) My neurologist agreed to stop my participation in the trial if it was severely affecting my health, but beyond that, I was never informed about what those tests revealed. I would estimate that for every minute I spent talking with my neurologist about my medical care, I spent ten hours in medical testing labs.

A resident guinea pig in places full of people who appeared overtly sick and debilitated, I often felt like an oddity. I felt similarly out of place in support groups. Some were composed of delightful, but older women with moderate to severe disability, whose lives and experiences were quite dissimilar from my own. Others were composed of predominately younger people who were mostly interested in keeping up with the latest medical breakthroughs. Medicine had taken up so much of my time and energy that I found little interest in exhausting myself any further on the enterprise. One group I attended went by the acronym H.O.P or "Happy Optimistic People," which was reason enough to never go again. I am all for defying the cultural expectation that people with chronic illness are tragic and sad, but demanding that they be happy instead seems nearly as oppressive. Our culture places many demands and expectations on the chronically ill and disabled.

Naturally, physicians have been highly prescriptive in their evaluation of my illness. In the months and years following my diagnosis, my neurologists frequently commented upon my seeming healthiness, only to remind me that patients tend to do well in their first five years after diagnosis. I am not sure if they were attempting to prepare me for a possible reversal of my fortunes, but the statement always felt insensitive and presumptuous. Never once has a neurologist asked me about my diet or exercise routines or how I imagine I would cope with a disability. Now, when my neurologists comment on my health and strength, they attribute it to the wonderful (now FDA-approved!) drugs I am taking.

After meeting me for the first time, one neurologist declared, "You appear to be in good health, that drug you take is really a wonder drug, isn't it?"

"I have no idea," I responded, "I have nothing to compare it to. It's the only MS medication I have ever taken and I feel the same as before I started taking it." He appeared unsure how to respond. To restore his faith in medicine, perhaps I should have added that, unlike some other users of the drug, I didn't immediately die of heart failure after taking my first dose, so I have really come out on top in that respect. I have met older and even elderly women with MS who have no visible signs of the disease, and they went the majority of their lives without any drugs at all. The disease is incredibly unpredictable, but in the face of uncertainty, my doctors are quick to credit medicine with the preservation of my bodily functioning. I have no intention of stopping my medication to test their theory, but I dislike the idea that any doctor would see my body as a primary example of the power of medicine.

LIVING IN ART

After my clinical trial ended, I was able to secure a modicum of distance from medicine's intrusion into my life, and I began to reflect more seriously on my ventures in the world of medicine. Sharing my reflections on the process of my medical imaging with my sister, we found that our personal and scholarly interests converged upon an unlikely common interest: Renaissance woodcuts. Darian had just begun her MFA in printmaking, and understanding the history of her craft was important for her development as an artist. She introduced me to Renaissance anatomical textbooks. Anatomical drawings, such as those in Andreas Vesalius' (1514–64) *De humani corporis fabrica*, depict bodies set within a theological backdrop that give the images rich meaning and context.[1] I could not help but note how different these depictions of the body were from the sterile illustrations I was accustomed to seeing in the images of my own body produced by medical imaging technology.

---

1. The following images are woodcuts after drawings attributed to Joannes Stephanus of Calcar (1499–c. 1546) from Vesalius, *De humani corporis fabrica libri septum* (Basel: Ioannis Oporini, 1543), 190, 201, and 246.

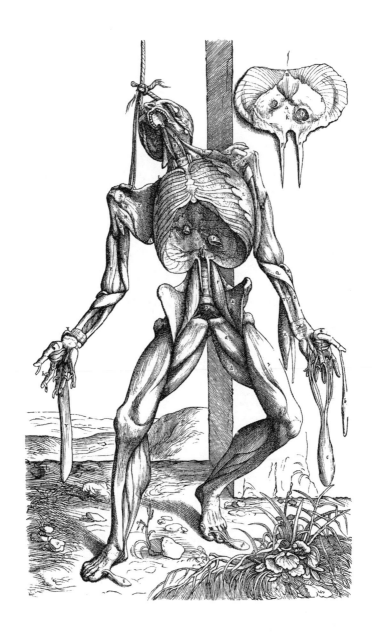

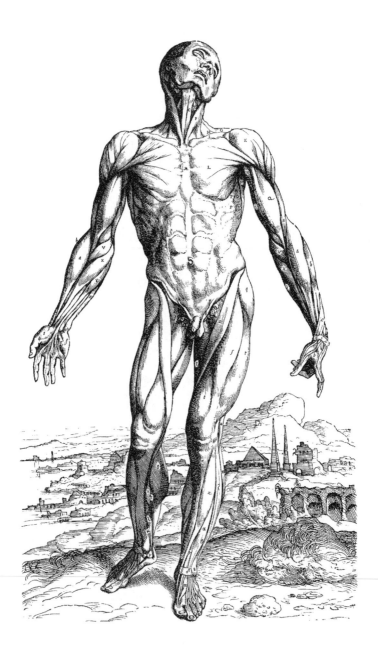

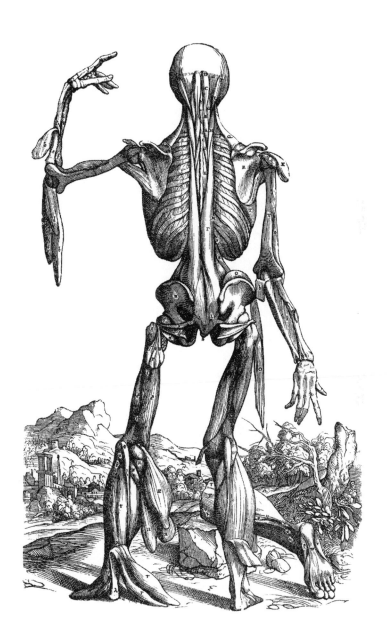

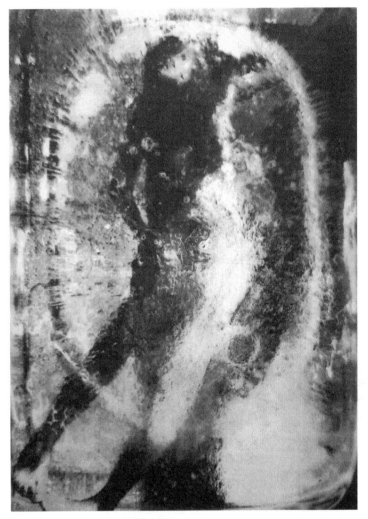

"Numb," Silkscreen, 40 x 32, 2013

The following Christmas, Darian presented me with a print she had made of my body. It is a beautiful depiction of a female figure frozen in ice, meant to convey the unreliable body experienced by people with MS. White spots float around the figure, recalling the lesions visible on my MRI scans. It was a lovely tribute to my ever-transforming body. Jokingly, I asked how she managed to get a nude photo of me without my knowledge. The body, of course, was hers, but it represented mine. The convergence of our bodies in print inspired another idea. Over the years, I had amassed thousands of MR images. The scanning process is such an uncomfortable one for me that I was determined that someone besides my physicians should benefit from the images produced. I procured a copy of my latest scans and sent them off to Darian, who was happy to examine them for artistic inspiration.

I also took time to peruse the images for myself, which I had never done before. I had seen my MR images many times, but always from behind my doctor's head in an exam room. On my own time and in the comfort of my own home, I saw the images in a new way. Given the callousness with which my first neurologist gazed upon my MR images and diagnosed me, I had never before felt the urge to examine them for myself. Now I was enthralled. I had not previously realized just how many images were produced during a single scanning session. With hundreds of images to pore over, I could now see the curve of my spinal column, the wrinkles in my brain, the protrusion of my eyes, a mash up of internal organs, and that layer of belly fat I am always trying to rid myself of. These images represented my body, some parts I was familiar with, while others appeared strange to me.

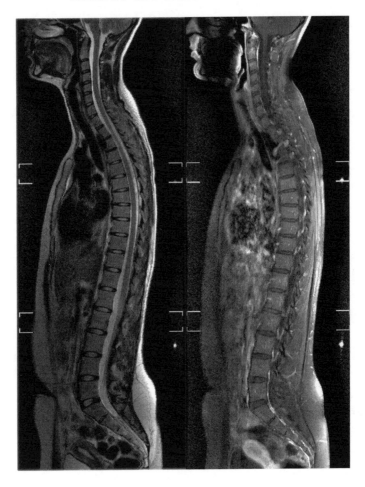

Darian's first reaction to the images was less appreciative, "You're a monster!" she declared. I did not notice at first, but she was right. Some of the images, particularly the ones that are angled down from top of my head, are a bit scary. I imagine as the older sister, this was not the first time I appeared scary to Darian. This image was one of me, but one that was hard to reconcile with the image of myself I am accustomed to seeing in the mirror. After my initial shock, I began to appreciate how the images captured various parts of my body and even evoked multiple aspects of my self-understanding.

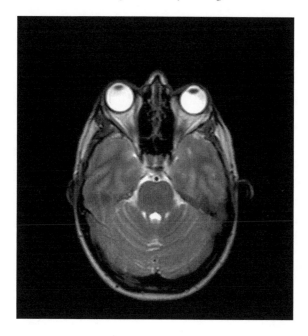

Over the past several years, Darian has been using my scans in her art. By re-presenting my scans in artistic form, she attempts to re-contextualize them. As a chronically ill person, I cannot completely escape the power medicine holds over me, but I can attempt to subvert its objectifying gaze and learn to see myself differently. I am more or less forced to allow my doctor to interpret my MR images, but I choose to allow Darian to have interpretive power as well. Giving Darian power over my body's representation has been both empowering and sometimes unnerving. As someone who truly who knows me (which admittedly includes the bad and good of me), she interprets my body with a fuller vision of who I am and the values that I hold. This is not to say, however, that she captures *me* in her prints. Her art both exceeds and limits my body. I am no more these images than I am a MRI scan, and at the same time, the images are more universal than I could ever hope to be. Through Darian's art, I learn to see myself differently and in multiplicity. I see myself becoming something new.

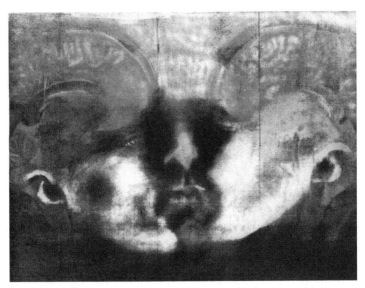

"The Scan and the Mirror," Stone lithography and silkscreen, 22" x 28," 2013

My diagnosis began with an image and now I am left wondering how I should see myself. Chronic illness now shapes my identity, but it leaves no visible scars. I am still learning how to live with illness, which I imagine to be a life-long process. I know that I am much more than my illness, but I also know that I cannot escape my illness by pretending that it is not a part of my life or that it does not shape my identity. I also know that because it is a progressive illness, living with MS will require constant readjustments. I no longer strive to acquire a stable body or identity; instead, I have come to value the becoming and unfolding of life, even though my unfolding is sometimes exasperating. The becoming of my life involves good days and bad, and I am not always sure which of my bodily failings are symptoms of a disease and which are simple missteps of a normally functioning body. My body remains partially mysterious, even to me. Multiple sclerosis continues to shape me in ways that I am perhaps only beginning to understand and in ways that I may never fully understand. Living in ambiguity can be frustrating, but I have little choice in the matter. There are, of course, worse things than giving up the illusory idea of complete control over one's fate. For now, I am learning how to live with the new images of myself I have acquired in the medical process, how to live with bodily ambiguity, and to how become disabled.

2

Lived Scans

Darian Goldin Stahl

I couldn't see *her*. Flipping through the thousands of grey and pixilated slices of this body on the computer screen, I could not recognize my own sister in a single image. I searched for the scans of her face. I finally found the file of images that scanned through Devan's skull from front to back. I immediately regretted seeking out these particular images as they made their way through her teeth and nasal cavity. Perhaps Devan could be shown in her eyes? No, she was not there either.

After my initial excitement of sifting through this new cache of imagery had worn off, I felt the injustice of them. These scans told Devan's doctors all they needed to know about her illness, but absolutely nothing about her. Her entire being has been reduced and quantified. Rather than hunt for the bright spots along her brain and spine that led to her diagnosis, I am drawn to the scans of her ear or cheek—useless for diagnostic purposes, but important to the loved one who seeks to recognize her sister's face. When I see these MRI scans, I imagine the hours she has spent in this cacophonous tube, trapped and still, and that her thoughts must wander to a future when she might always be still.

It was too painful to think about Devan's diagnosis in the beginning, and perhaps we didn't have to because we were not confronted with her MS. Since she always seemed "normal" and able, it was easy to choose not to think about her chronic illness and the abnormalities that grew inside the hidden depths of her anatomy. In our rather reserved military family, we chose the stiff-upper-lip approach of dealing with our pain. It took over four years for us to begin talking about Devan's diagnosis, a fact I am now ashamed to admit. I imagine she must have felt alone in these most vulnerable years, an isolation poignantly perpetuated by our family's acrobatic maneuvers to not talk about it.

The distance between formality and reality started to close when Devan sent me her articles for academic journals and conferences. Written from her unique point of view as a hospital chaplain, bioethics scholar, and patient, her words shed light on the lack of empathy for patients within the medical system from her first-person perspective. This was the first time I heard her talk about her disease. She revealed to me, along with all the other conference-goers, her diagnosis narrative and the powerlessness she felt when her tactless specialist pointed to bright spots between blurs of grey on his computer screen. I also felt powerless when reading her narratives. I felt a deep wrong was taking place when the doctors were more focused on the secretive results of the medical trials instead of helping my sister manage her symptoms and prepare for a life living with impairment. Her neurologist seemed to consider Devan as simply the sum of her scans. It pained me to think that a community of healers could see her only as a fractured self. But then again, in my shortsighted attempts to make everything seem fine, I was also ignoring a part of her new and changing identity as a woman with disease.

It was during these initial years of my sister's illness that I was becoming a printmaker. After falling in love with the medium during my study abroad in Venice, Italy, I continued to learn more about the history of printmaking in a course on anatomy in the Renaissance. I was struck by the illustrators' ability to inform the viewer of their philosophical beliefs by employing the body as a metaphorical vehicle. The positioning of the hands, an upward gaze, or the elegance of the figure all served to perpetuate the belief of humanity's dominion on earth. By further depicting the anatomical figure within an environment, the artists and anatomists situated medical imagery within their contemporary real-world contexts. This rich and layered imagery is in stark contrast to the sterile, anonymous, even genderless medical images of today. In many ways, the grotesque, bloody, flayed bodies depicted in the Renaissance woodcuts better articulate a real confrontation with the human form than contemporary medical imaging techniques. In discussion over this shared interest, Devan and I came to the conclusion that if modern scans included context and evidence of the patient's life, they would possess more potential for empathy creation between doctors and patients. They could remind the viewers that medical scans represent the flesh, bones, and sinew of a real, whole person. This conversation gave me a new goal for my printmaking: create medical images within a context that spoke about the lived experiences of Devan Stahl.

The goals of this project are twofold. First, I can continue to discuss and unpack the emotions around Devan's diagnosis and repair the damage that silence has inflicted on our family. Second, this research-creation project has the potential to impact other patients as well, and leave a lasting impression on the burgeoning field of medical humanities. My work is now motivated by the desire to understand how our sense of self has been transformed as a result of our entanglements with biomedical imaging technologies. It is also guided by the ethical desire to instigate meaningful collaborations with those whose subjectivities are being shaped by the experience of illness; and finally to see what role aesthetics can play to foster interdisciplinary collaborations between art and medicine. By re-contextualizing her medical scans through a fine-art lens that humanizes their alienating qualities, I aim to restore Devan's sense of agency over her medicalized body.

So far, the print-based artwork I have created combines my sister's MRI scans with domestic spaces to represent the uneasy relationship between a likely future of impairment and continuing her daily life in the present. Although these prints are specifically about my sister, the work is open enough for a multiplicity of meaning for individual viewers. I feel compelled to create this work because Devan is brave enough to share her writings as a way to process personal feelings and act as a bridge between the biomedical and patient communities. Perhaps I can likewise use my artistic ability to express her experiences, and in some way, show her my empathy.

RESEARCH-CREATION

This research-creation project is a collaborative cycle of informing and reconstructing illness identity, with the aim of advancing the field of medical humanities and fostering a more empathetic relationship between medical practitioners and their patients. Because there are multiple ways of learning and knowing, I found that realizing Devan's narratives visually through research-creation would complement and add insight to her writing. My ambition is always to elicit tacit learning of the chronically ill patient through an honest portrayal of living with disease in ways writing cannot. For my first gesture toward an embodied creation, I began freezing small images of the nude figure in blocks of ice as a metaphor for the neuropathy and numbness that is symptomatic of MS. I also chose to depict large, floating, bright spots over the figure's head, a visual language reminiscent of thought bubbles, but which also recall the bright abnormalities in her scans. I thought of this figure as thinking ahead to a future with numbness and impairment. Although I used my own body for the figure, she is meant to be Devan. This initial act of our bodies and intention coming together to create a metaphorical figure situated in the center of our partnership opened the door to a more complete bodily collaborative practice.

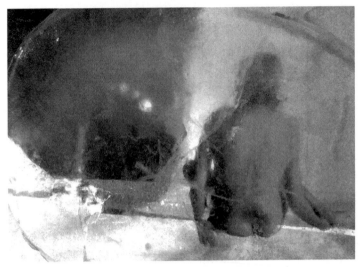

"Frozen," Silkscreen, 32" x 36," 2013

A breakthrough in our collaboration to give context to the medicalized body came when Devan procured her MRI scans from her doctors so that I could incorporate them into my artwork. This was the first time she had seen her scans outside of the doctor's office, and the first time I had ever seen them. We now had time and privacy to contemplate these powerful images. After many viewings, I found that even these abstracted reductions of my sister's body held clues and insights into the process of being scanned. I was first struck by the amount of images. There were thousands slices going from top to bottom, front to back, and side to side.

Some scans showed her body lit with injected contrast, and others were dark. Some bodies were crisp and clear, while others were blurry. I can imagine the despair she must have felt when the doctors told her she did not keep still well enough, and they would have to repeat the process again. The time spent in this cacophonous tube is daunting.

I then became very interested in the groups of text on the four corners of every scanned image. As a printmaker, I am well versed in the use of text and image. The text presented in these scans, however, only served to confuse the image instead of adding clarity. They are medical codes, vitally important to the doctor's specialized knowledge I am sure, but elucidated how very little I know about the scanning technology. The codes supply the ultimate quantification of the body revealed in the scans. It made me uncomfortable to think that these reduced scanned images could be even further abstracted until the whole body was simply a stunted grouping of numbers and letters. Devan's name and date of birth are also in the corner of every slide, but even this small bit of information utterly fails to give any identifying meaning to these stiff, gray, blurry images, and could not be further from how I see Devan.

Armed with these MRI scans and Devan's narratives on living with illness, I sought to re-contextualize her medicalized body and present a nuanced image of what it is like to live with a diagnosis of chronic illness. At first, I was at a loss about how these stiff, pixilated, and eerie images related to my sister's lived experiences. Although the current symptoms of her MS are generally controlled, the looming potential and progressive loss of proprioception is a deep concern. Like my first gesture to impart a visual context to Devan's illness, I chose an image of Devan's spine to print and freeze in ice. This time, however, I chose to set her MRI within a glass mason jar: a vessel to act as her metaphorical body. This glass home is at once strong and useful, with ties to traditional women's work, but also brittle and even dangerous under stress. I placed the spine within the jar, filled it with water, and left it outside in a bitterly cold Canadian winter's night. While sleeping, the ice had expanded and shattered its glass skin, but the freezing temperatures were holding every piece in place. Careful not to cut my hands on the shards, I took my dangerous vessel inside and created a time-lapse video of the jar melting over the next sixteen hours. The splinters of glass fell away and shattered on the ground, the melting ice dripped off its shrinking body, and finally, the spine crumpled down with no more frozen viscera to support it. When I present this footage, I play this small drama in reverse before it begins again. The mess of scan, shards, and water are reconstituted to their original form—never wholly unbroken, but standing. I see the reversal and continuous loop of melting and freezing as the relapse and remission cycle of MS.

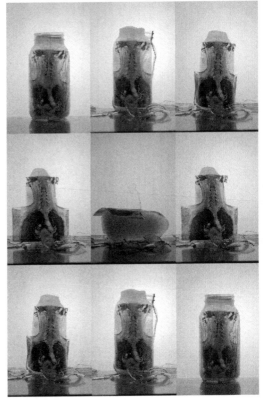

"Relapse/Remission," Time-lapse video stills, 00:05:10, 2015

Like Vesalius' anatomical figures, I also yearned to set Devan's scans within a contemporary, everyday context. I wanted to create a phenomenological encounter with these scans that normally exist in a purely digital space, because there is a tension between what doctors say exists within her brain and what she is able to perceive. I thought that if she were able to touch her interior self, perhaps she could relate in a tactile way to the disease that resides there. After many failed attempts to photographically or drawerly merge the scans with the exterior body, I discovered a way of "scanning" my own skin. By pressing my body into charcoaled paper, I am able to leave a negative impression of my skin with incredible detail. The creases of my lips, hairs on my cheek, and even the pores of my chin are all impressed on the paper in crisp precision. The charcoal itself adds a black depth and frame to the image that is reminiscent of the original MRI scans. I now had the beginnings of a visual language I could employ to join the digital body with a phenomenological encounter. By layering the interior body with the surface impressions through the printmaking process, I am creating a metaphorical figure that cannot hide away from her disease because she wears the evidence of it on her skin.

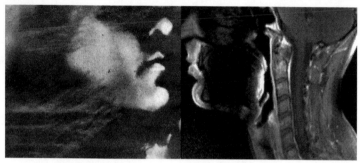

"Skin and Scan," Charcoal and MRI scan, 10" x 24," 2013

Rather than simply layering these two images in an aesthetic manner, I sought to portray the lived experiences of moving through the world with disease. I began to imagine moments when she agonizes over her scans so intensely, that the scans push and manifest themselves onto the surface. What came to mind was the shared experience we all must have of lying in bed, unable to fall asleep due to anxiety. We toss and turn, searching for rest but unable to shirk off the worry. With this intention in mind, I attempted to capture surface scans of the restless body on large sheets of charcoaled paper. Wearing my pajamas and thinking about the positions I am able to fall asleep in, I carefully rolled my body over long sheets of dark paper. The oils in my skin, the texture of my hair, and the cloth of my shirt all lift the charcoal and reveal a grotesque and pulled-apart body. She is morphing through the composition as a mass of arms and faces. This figure becomes a metaphorical agent for the tension she feels with her body. I subtly layered the MRI scans in an attempt to fit them onto this monstrous woman, to give some clue to the viewer of what plagues her mind during this restless night.

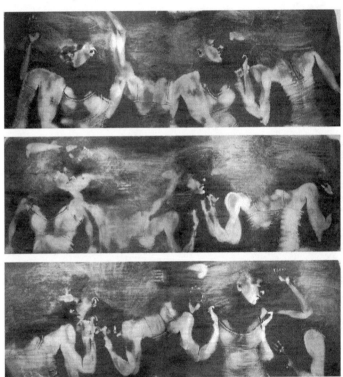

"Restless," Archival inkjet print on film, 96" x 88," 2014

The figures in this image are printed to the body's size, and the full piece stands at almost 9 feet high and 8 feet across. My intent in printing at this scale was to create a looming and daunting portrait that confronts the viewer. Like a filmstrip, the repetition of the figure through three horizontal planes gives a sense of time to the piece, suggesting a durational unease. The image is also printed on film, to recall the original MRI substrate. Finally, the repetitious, cinematic quality of this piece relates to the viewer the inescapable echo of what plagues her thoughts at night.

Since Devan is not yet experiencing disability on a daily basis, it might be easy to fall into the routine of living and not dwelling on her unreliable body. There are short but heavy moments, however, that interrupt the routine of life, when she is once again reminded of her disease. These instances happen when a tangible experience affects psychological spaces, such as dropping keys in the foyer or tripping on the corner of a rug. Is she just being clumsy, or is she having a relapse? Being forcibly *reminded* of disease has stuck with me. In this moment of uncertainty, the scanned and lived worlds collide and she is momentarily caught immobile between them.

I was also caught unaware one morning when the lights from between the Venetian blinds of my bedroom glowed brightly on the opposite walls. This perfectly common occurrence took on a completely new context after viewing Devan's MRI scans. The columns of light arrested me, as they utterly mirrored the spinal column exposed in her scans. Whereas only the brightest spots in Devan's scans reveal the lesions, this spine in my apartment shone fully bright. Perhaps I was glimpsing a scan from the future where the lesions fully conquer her nerves. How perversely they crept around my living room walls, haunting my thoughts for days afterwards. I began following and photographing them every morning. These light columns became another way of joining the scanned and lived worlds, and became the next layer in my prints.

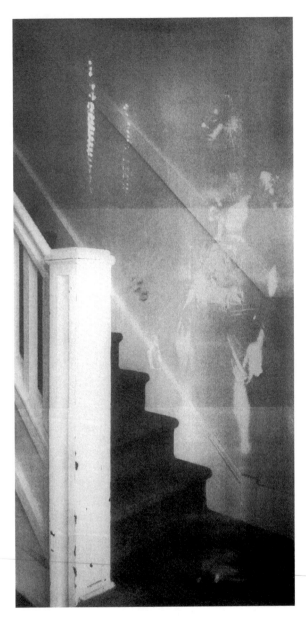

"Stairway," Silkscreen, 84" x 42," 2014

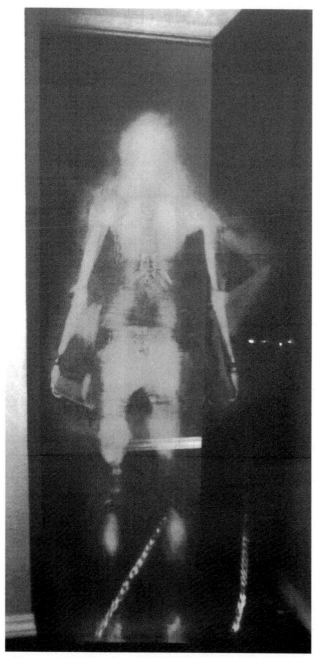

"Doorway," Silkscreen, 84" x 42," 2013

This new figure, the proxy for my sister, her narratives, and our collaborative process, is not confined to seas of gray and the black frame of a computer screen. This agent can go home. Whereas the digital body was housed in the clinic, I choose to depict our proxy in domestic spaces. This housing is meant to situate her within the daily life of a person who lives with a diagnosis.

Our proxy is depicted at the base of stairs or in narrow doorways—places she might not always be able to navigate as neuropathy creeps up her legs. She cannot feel the lesions, but has an intuitive sense of them. They are an invisible stress that she carries with her, hidden from society and felt only by the burden on her soul from the knowledge of what grows within. For our proxy, the psychological weight of waiting for impairment is worn on her ghostly skin as she gazes toward the viewer in a charged silence.

I chose to depict the moment of colliding exterior and interior realms in a life-sized photographic print so that a full confrontation with another body can occur. These prints are a full-body surface impression of my exterior joined with Devan's MRI scans, and includes a view of two rooms joined by the spine of light. My aim was to give the viewers a sense of concrete space that, perhaps, they too might occupy one day. In these prints, the bodily fantasy of a glowing and voracious disease is fully formed. In the moment when the light shines through the window of her apartment, the figure identifies wholly with the diseased part of herself and becomes a scan entirely. The body diffuses and is fixed haunting the domestic spaces that troubled her most in life.

BOOK WORKS

Something that is missing in the previous printwork was the literal voice of Devan. I wanted to give her the opportunity to express her unease to the viewer. If I found such rich insight and inspiration in her writing, perhaps others could as well. My first investigation into an Artist Book that inhabits Devan's experiences is called "The Importance of Dualism." This title was taken from a journal entry Devan wrote that recounts her diagnosis narrative and conveys how it felt to see her MRI scans for the first time. This bookwork concentrates on the complex emotions that accompany a medical diagnosis of chronic illness and the status of our fallible bodies. I am most interested in the psychological schism between what the body is able to perceive and what is revealed by internal medical scans. I aim to restore this fractured sense of identity by joining Devan's voice with her medical scans to re-humanize their anonymous and alienating qualities.

I began by layering Devan's text over her MRI scans. Next, I used the printmaking method photo-intaglio to print the plates onto incredibly thin Japanese silk tissue paper using dark blue ink. The final pages are then dipped into beeswax to render them translucent and imbue the paper with an eerie skin-like quality. Finally, the binding of the book recalls medical stitches, which alludes to the conflict she feels with her interior body.

The MRI machine stacks exceptionally thin slices of my sister's inner anatomy for the doctors to sift through. Likewise, the viewers of this bodily book flip through her scans and narrative on fine, transparent pages. The buildup of imagery and words seen through the pages point to the overwhelming amount of uneasy thoughts that come in a moment of diagnosis. This expression of our partnership holds her narrative, internal anatomy, and skin's surface together for the first time. Our voices combine through printmaking to construct this book, which is the amalgamation of our collaborative endeavors to give context to the medicalized body.

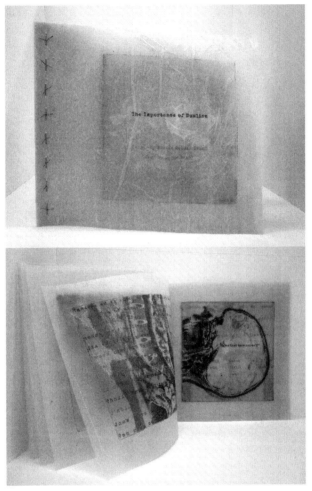

"The Importance of Dualism," Photo-intaglio and encaustic, 9" x 10," 2014

My next bookwork focuses on living with the weight of a diagnosis in everyday life. By combining the patterns found on hospital gowns, MRI scans, as well as patterns found in the home, I aim to give a more holistic view of what it is like to live with disease beyond the hospital doors.

I developed a toner-transfer technique that allows me to print onto waxed silk. The ultra-fine silk pages are first dipped into pigmented encaustic wax. Next, my image is physically pressed into the surface of the wax, which is able to hold the toner. Because toner is a plastic, and plastic can dissolve in an oil, the image adheres to the wax surface of each page after intensive burnishing. This process allows me to incorporate a full-color range and control for the opacity or transparency of each page, all while keeping the flexibility and translucency of silk. Finally, the pages are bound using a stab stitch that recalls the spinal column portrayed in the book.

The book is housed in a plexiglass box that is reminiscent of the hospital's red "MRI IN USE" light box signs. The text is a first-person narrative from my sister, while she reflects on her experiences in the hospital. Each letter in the text has been appropriated from the metadata in her MRI scans, and arranged in the same encoded and confusing manner. This gesture forces a slower read, while both the viewer and my sister must decipher difficult memories. The images combine her MRI scans, hospital gowns, and the horizontal lines that are produced from light escaping between Venetian blinds. This mix of medical imagery and home produce a psychological snapshot of the patient's uneasy mind while she is being scanned, and how these memories then follow her through daily life.

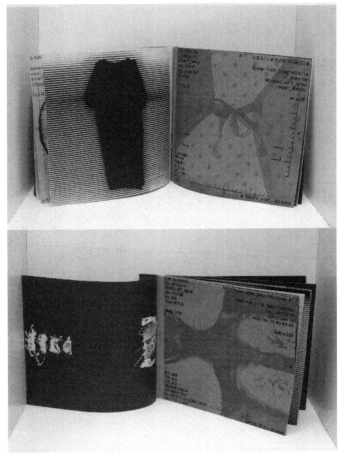

"MRI IN USE," Encaustic toner transfer on silk, 8" x 9.5," 2015

CONCLUSION

The works presented in this chapter are a part of the continuing pursuit to reclaim, re-present, and identify with the ill body. While MRI scans reveal truths about the patient's body, they cannot speak to what it is like moving through our world with chronic illness. By engaging in an artistic reclamation over medical imagery, I seek to better reveal this all-too human experience.

The journey from patient to print is an act of many translations. First, the real, fleshy, and leaky body is severely transcribed by penetrating waves of magnetic resonance. All meaning of the person is lost, notwithstanding the reason for the scan: a readable diagnosis. Although the consequences of viewing one's own scanned body follows the patient well beyond the hospital doors, this sterile space is generally the only time the patient views their scans—forever cementing the memory of the medicalized body with the anxiety of diagnosis. By reclaiming the scanned body from the doctor's specialized knowledge, I am translating the body once again. With each layer in the printmaking process, I am encoding and decoding context and lived experiences. Although I could never hope to create an image that fully and irreducibly represents Devan, the act of giving skin back to her scans and sending them home is my way of imbuing multitudes into the singular purpose of the MR image.

The final translation of the body occurs in the perpetually negotiated space between the print and the viewer, when the image is internalized and imbued with meaning from each person's situated knowledge. Although this work is specifically about my sister and her contemplations over her prognosis, disability is a universal condition that all too often is shunned away and ignored. Therein lies the paradox of disability art: if the artwork is too explicit about disability, a barrier can occur if its audience can no longer be critical of the work; but if the image is too universal, it ceases to be about the lived experience of disability. To navigate this space between alienation and ambiguity, I strive to create honest work on the subject of disability, but leave the images open enough for multiple interpretations.

This artwork also inhabits a space between arts and science. The medical humanities give scientists the opportunity to step back and consider the larger, intangible implications of their research, such as the psychological impact of viewing one's internal disease. Scientific research is goal- and results-oriented, and only a few of the thousands of MRI scans are valuable for diagnostic purposes. As an artist, however, I am much more interested in investigating how these scans affect the patient they are meant to represent. My research-creation asks how a phenomenological encounter with their internal medical scans can impact a patient's sense of identity and agency and, in turn, change the way a doctor views her patient from a representative object into irreducible subject. My goal is not only to discover what medical technologies can offer an artist, but also how art can impact those medical practitioners. Finally, I aim to show how interdisciplinary research-creation can allow for an empathetic exchange between an ableist society and those who live with bodily unease or impairment.

I strive to create empathy for the un-well body by visualizing the patient narrative. Through the layering of MRI technology, ghostly skin impressions, and images of the home, I am able to contextualize internal medical scans within the patient's daily experiences with illness. It is a performative and subversive act to re-present internal medical scans through an embodied fine-art lens, for what is not seen in these highly stylized and pixilated MRI scans is the very human experience of living with chronic illness day after day. Building on the premise of narrative, my artwork will continue to address the immense issues surrounding the ill body, with the ultimate aim of building a productive dialogue within the medical community on the complexities and (often) distress of the patient experience.

The arts-based research I present is not a final answer or an end, but an interdisciplinary untangling of social issues that advances the burgeoning field of medical humanities. Unlike a doctor, I am not interested in pointing to diagnosable areas of the MRI scans. Instead, I use the scans as a visual metaphor for living with bodily un-ease. Although this work is about multiple sclerosis in particular, the artwork is open enough for viewers to impart their own identity and experiences within the medical system, and come to find we all carry anxiety about our bodies and, more broadly, our mortality. Identification with differing bodies is what ignites the empathetic exchange between able and impaired peoples. My aim is not to "celebrate" or "fight" difference, but to foster an ethical turn in medicine and greater society where difference is expected and respected.

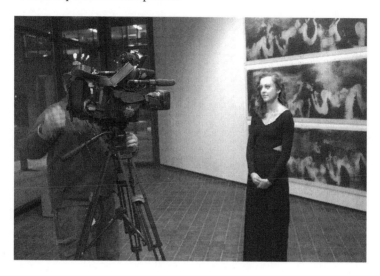

3

"The becoming of my life . . . ":
Liminality, Pathography, and Identity

THERESE JONES

> This is the important point about the stories we tell our-
> selves about our lives: We make them up as we go along.
> We can't select every event and detail, of course. We can't
> decide, for instance, whether or not someone gets MS.
> MS just *happens*. But—and this is the exciting part—we
> can choose how we will respond to that happening, what
> kind of role we will give it in the story we're making up
> as we go along.[1]

IN MEDIA RES

There is no "going along" at the beginning of Devan Stahl's narrative of multiple sclerosis, "Living into My Image." There is
no going anywhere at all given that she is immobilized in what

1. Mairs, *Carnal Acts: Essays*, 124.

42

she calls the dark narrow tunnel of an MRI scanner. This physical confinement is mirrored by a kind of existential entrapment—being compelled to give consent, to "subject" herself to a procedure that she describes as one in which her whole body feels like it will rip apart. While she duly acknowledges that she is a "willing participant," that she has "agreed to be in the scanner" and has "agreed that it was best for [her] health," she consistently undermines these professions or protestations of autonomy with the repeated use of the word *force* and with descriptions of being in a "vulnerable position" and being unable to escape. She acts, willingly and unwillingly, in order to be acted upon.

From the outset, both reader and narrator find themselves in the middle of things. For the reader, the story unfolds somewhere and sometime in what appears to be a biomedical event. We know that something has happened but not what it is; we have neither context nor causality. Our narrator is literally imprisoned in a tube, figuratively affixed like a specimen on a slide or detained like a person of interest. By the second paragraph, however, we learn the nature of her problem (or offense): she is "chronically ill" and thus, requires "constant monitoring."

For the narrator, the opening scene provides an opportunity to pause and consider not only what has happened to her but also who she is and who she will become. The question of identity—how it is hijacked by chronic illness—is at the core of Stahl's story, and it is fitting that she employs the familiar poetic device of *in media res*, long used to draw back the curtain on the journey of an epic hero in search of self.

Traversing through the analytic frames of social anthropology and socio-narratology, this chapter approaches Stahl's personal account of MS as an experience of liminality—a state that Victor Turner describes as interstructural or betwixt and between—as well as an elaboration of how narrative simultaneously captures and creates meaning for individuals who experience disrupted lives and "shattered" identities (to use Stahl's own words) from chronic illness. I begin with a general discussion of liminality, which is especially helpful in understanding the dynamic process of alienation and adaptation that accompanies the diagnosis of serious or chronic illness and that grounds it in the fact of its embodiment. This is particularly relevant to Stahl's account as she tries to express the confusion of being labeled as ill but appearing (and feeling) healthy.

Following from that discussion, I will turn to pathography. Such stories of sickness often reveal a person's conception of how identity is constructed—both its process of development as well as its essential attributes. Arthur Frank writes that stories themselves perform the work of subjectification: "they are subjectifiers, telling people who they ought to be, who they might like to be and who they can be."[2] For Stahl, a young adult only recently exploring the possibilities of career, questioning her own and others' beliefs and values, and coming to accept and appreciate her woman's body, the diagnosis of MS renders her mute and unrecognizable: "I have no more questions. I am empty. . . . The diagnosis began with an image, and now I am left wondering how I should see myself. Chronic illness shapes my identity, but it leaves no scars."[3]

Finally, in the last section of this chapter, I will expand the discussion of narrative as Stahl struggles not only to recover her voice but also to discover a way of resisting and ultimately transforming the biomedical determination of what counts as sick and not sick and how that determination serves as an organizing principle of knowing ourselves as healthy or unhealthy. One of the great perceptions of Michel Foucault is that the self's sense of its health *within* derives from *outside* the body.[4] It is stories, Cheryl Mattingly argues, that challenge the hegemony of structural accounts—such as the notion that life follows a predictable arc or that illness is an aberration to be engineered out of existence—by highlighting "the unfinished, idiosyncratic, unpredictable, suspenseful qualities . . . that reveal the exigencies of human temporality and the contingencies of social life . . . ."[5] It is when Stahl not only accepts but

2. Frank, "Health Stories as Connectors and Subjectifiers," 430.

3. Stahl, "Living into My Image," 1–17, in this volume.

4. Frank, "Health Stories as Connectors and Subjectifiers," 424.

5. Mattingly, *The Paradox of Hope*, 42–43.

also embraces the ambiguity of life *and* irreducibility of the body that she breaks away from the silence and stasis effected by the diagnostic moment—"It's MS!"—and moves toward the generative and interpretive possibilities of narrative—"I can . . . learn to see myself differently."[6]

ON LIMINALITY

> Imagine a life in which feasible others—others you can hope to be like—don't exist[:] . . . you might conclude that there is something queer about you, something ugly or foolish or shameful, . . . you might feel as though you don't exist, in any meaningful social sense, at all.[7]

Liminal and liminality (derived from the Latin, *limen,* meaning "threshold") were introduced to anthropology in 1909 by Arnold Van Gennep in his work on the rites of passage that accompany every change of place, state, position, and age and are marked by three phases:

- *separation* in which a person is stripped of status and detached from the social structure

- *limen* in which a passenger enters an ambiguous period of transition

- *aggregation* in which a subject is given a new status.[8]

In the second half of the twentieth century, Victor Turner borrowed and expanded Van Gennep's concept of liminality, thereby ensuring widespread use of it in anthropology and other fields such as performance studies and neuropsychology. Turner initially formulates the theory in a chapter, "Betwixt and Between: The Liminal Period in *Rites de Passage,*" defining states as "relatively fixed or stable conditions" and characterizing the transitions

6. Stahl, "Living into My Image," 16.

7. Mairs, *Carnal Acts: Essays,* 33–34.

8. Van Gennep, *The Rites of Passage,* 21.

between them as "a process, a becoming, [and] a transformation."[9] Thus, the qualities of liminality are necessarily ambiguous and marginal, as persons slip through or by the networks of classifications that normally locate states and positions in cultural space. Two years later, Turner elaborates the "being and nothingness" of liminal persons or "threshold people" in the context of everyday life, noting that their passivity and malleability are the externalization of a process in which they are ground down, refashioned, and endowed with new powers to cope going forward.[10]

These rites of passage with their betwixt and between-ness, their indeterminate and inferior qualities of liminality, have been used as a heuristic model with which to understand and explain the changes that result during experiences of serious or chronic illness. In that context, several formulations of liminality are offered. For example, Arthur Kleinman documents the sense of apartness with particular clarity in which certain labels "encase the patient in a visible exoskeleton of powerfully peculiar meanings that the patient must deal with, as must those of us who are around the patient."[11] In *The Absent Body*, Drew Leder recognizes that coming to an awareness of the body is alienating and incommunicable to someone who has not shared the experience.[12] In her discussion of chronic illness, Kathy Charmaz explores how the silences, false starts, and fragmented expressions so typical of the disruption of illness enact how "liminal identity questions may erode taken-for-granted images of self" and how the liminal experience "feels strange, alien, apart from life."[13] And in narrative accounts, liminality has served as a way to describe an ill person's abandonment of structure and routine.[14]

Arguably, the most thorough and thoughtful exploration of liminality is the analysis and discussion by Little et al. who studied

---

9. Turner, *The Forest of Symbols*, 93–94.

10. Turner, *The Ritual Process*, 1969.

11. Kleinmann, *The Illness Narratives*, 22.

12. Leder, *The Absent Body*.

13. Charmaz, "Stories and Silences," 303–10.

14. Frankenberg, "Sickness as a Cultural Performance," 603–26.

both clinical cases and personal narratives as well as conducted interviews with people who had been diagnosed and treated for cancer.[15] They make two significant contributions to the understanding of liminality as a major category of illness experience: first, that any serious and chronic illness is, *itself,* a process of liminality which persists for the rest of a patient's life and second, that there are three major themes that emerge when patients recount the subjective experiences of symptoms, diagnosis, and treatment.

Stahl's narrative, for instance, exemplifies what the authors describe as the immediate and acute phase of liminality, which follows upon the diagnosis of a serious or chronic illness: "I am left wondering how I should see myself."[16] Her subsequent awareness if not acceptance of what she apprehends as the "life-long process" of learning how to live with illness is also representative of the enduring and sustained phase of liminality, the mode of life in which Stahl now inhabits and which she describes as mysterious, ambiguous, unstable, and exasperating. The authors emphasize how the liminal life is also the existential life in which the person must not only confront "the dread of the nothing into which we apparently go" but also live "separated from other lives . . . by the symptoms and disabilities of the illness."[17] This insight is borne out in Stahl's account of seeing herself "differently and in multiplicity"; of making "constant readjustments"; and of "giving up the illusory idea of complete control over one's fate."

In all of the narratives they analyze, Little and colleagues find three consistent responses to illness, what they call themes:

- *Patientness*: the persistent identification as a patient regardless of the presence or absence of disease.

- *Communicative alienation*: the state of alienation from others because of an inability to communicate and share the experience.

15. Little et al., "Liminality," 1485–94.
16. Stahl, "Living into My Image," 20.
17. Little et al. "Liminality," 1490.

47

- *Boundedness:* the awareness of a contracted and limited sense of space, time, and empowerment.[18]

Stahl's narrative includes all three themes, with the most explicit and dramatic examples tumbling throughout her account of the days after the initial diagnosis of MS. For example, she poses a series of rather panicky questions which express the boundedness that patients most often represent as loss of personal autonomy, self-determination, social identity, and a future: "Illness and disability would surely make me weak and make my goals in life . . . harder to achieve than ever. What if I couldn't walk? What if I went blind? What if I lost my memory and couldn't be a scholar? Will anyone ever want to marry me or have children with me?"[19]

She also expresses the challenge of trying to accept and accommodate a new status and a new role—that of patient. Little et al. note a range of responses to patientness: from disbelief to confusion to urgency to recognition that special strengths and personal resources must be marshalled.[20] Stahl describes a tension between her resistance to the totalizing identity of patient and her awareness that others expect her to behave as one:

> . . . my illness has become such a large part of my identity that I cannot hide it away. But it's never easy. People always expect you to be sad or strong about it. They want you to fight it and keep it distant from yourself . . . to persevere . . . to be quiet about it . . . . For me, constantly battling or pitying my own body feels like an exhausting snare of self-loathing.[21]

Finally, it is the theme of communication alienation that is most prominent in Stahl's narrative and most illustrative of the separateness and inchoateness of liminality. Beginning with her speechless reaction to the diagnosis of MS, her silences as often as her words signify an embodied subjectivity that represents the

18. Ibid., 1486–88.
19. Stahl, "Living into My Image," 8.
20. Little et al., "Liminality," 1486.
21. Stahl, "Living into My Image," 8.

fluidity of health and illness as well as the effacement of being labeled as disabled. For example, there is the moment following diagnosis in which she cannot speak—"I had no voice for it yet."[22] In her work on liminality, Cindy Mendelson writes that diagnosis often precipitates a loss of identity and induces a period of ambiguity in which the woman is not who she was.[23] Such loss is literally borne out with Stahl's inability to say what "it" is or what "it" means to her. Following this is her account of an exchange in which she will not speak—"What came out of my mouth was an unsettling period of silence" followed by "incomprehensible words of explanation"—because she feels "forced to explain the diagnosis" in order to receive financial support from the university. Here she resists constructing a purposeful and persuasive story of calamity and exigency, a common strategy for people with chronic illness in order to "keep their suffering out of view" and to "manage difficult people or situations."[24]

Yet, the fact of the narrative itself—the attempt at a rational ordering of experience—testifies to Stahl's hope of transcending or at least managing the alienation and incoherence of a disrupted life. Frank points out that the illness story faces a dual task: it must "restore an order that the interruption fragmented" yet "tell the truth that the interruptions will continue."[25] Stahl's movements between articulation and muteness perform this seemingly contradictory work by relating through language those moments when she is unable or unwilling to speak her suffering, to make sense of the unpredictable, overwhelming, and indescribable body.

22. Ibid., 8.
23. Mendelson, "Diagnosis," 391.
24. Charmaz, "Stories and Silences," 308.
25. Frank, *The Wounded Story Teller*, 59.

ON PATHOGRAPHY

> If we find the work of utterance getting easy or univer-
> sally acceptable, we're probably not doing it right.[26]

The liminality of illness experience is both reflected in and resisted through narrative. This tension is most evident in the shifting patterns and multiple versions of the story itself. In his ground-breaking work on pathography, *The Wounded Storyteller*, Frank emphasizes how becoming seriously ill is a call for stories because "stories have to *repair* the damage that illness has done to the ill person's sense of where she is in life, and where she may be going" as well as serve as accounts for family members, friends, health professionals, and even university registrars about what may or may not be going on.[27] Thus, illness narratives can be viewed as a dynamic process of constructing and reconstructing stories of embodied experience for both teller and listener. Moreover, their very composition—their alternating and overlapping structures—can signify the particularity of an experience as well as exhibit cultural and personal preferences.

In order to identify compositional threads and competing preferences, Frank proposes three types of narratives, all told alter-natively and repeatedly during illness, and all represented in Stahl's account.[28] For instance, the most common plotline—the "restitution narrative"—is structured linearly with comprehensible cause and effect: it begins with illness and ends with health. This type is familiar because we most often tell it ourselves and most often hear it told in media and medicine. It is, as Frank notes, "the cultur-ally preferred narrative,"[29] and Stahl's recognition that her doctors are "quick to credit medicine with the preservation of [her] bodily functioning"[30] without considering either the disease's unpredict-

---

26. Mairs, *Carnal Acts: Essays*, 63.
27. Frank, *The Wounded Storyteller*, 53. Emphasis in original.
28. Ibid., 76–77.
29. Ibid., 83.
30. Stahl, "Living into My Image," 11.

ability or the patient's healthy regimen of diet and exercise exemplifies biomedicine's preference for this narrative type. For Stahl herself, the moment of diagnosis with its stutter of questions about causation and responsibility ("How could he tell? Didn't I see this coming? Didn't I do an Internet search on this? Were [the other doctors] lying? Did they know? Did they suspect?") effectively undermines any hope of constructing a restitution narrative no matter how desirable its romantic structure of sickness, remedy, and restoration of health: "I cannot escape my illness . . . ," she writes.[31]

Chaos narratives are the opposite of restitution narratives, even *anti-narratives*: "time without sequence, telling without mediation, and speaking about oneself without fully able to reflect on oneself."[32] One prominent feature of the chaos narrative is a loss of control. Stahl repeats the words *forced* and *vulnerable* at the opening of her narrative to express both the literal and existential paralysis of being chronically ill and constantly monitored. The dehumanization of the medical gaze is compounded by the objectification of the male gaze in her rambling account of an older male radiology technician who first questions her about her bra and next comments about how some women might enjoy the vibration of an MRI scanner. In trying to make sense of this encounter, Stahl herself recognizes how confused, how "counterintuitive," she sounds when she first advises readers to leave on their clothes and next cautions them about "perverted old men [who] convince you *not* to take your clothes off," lest you miss the thrill of the exam.[33] The anecdote expresses both the murky predicament of a chaos story wrapped around the damaging illogic of sexual victimization: whatever she does or doesn't do, she is at risk; she is somehow responsible; yet she has no control.

While restitution stories attempt to render illness transitory and fix-able, chaos stories reveal contingency and uncertainty, especially relevant to the experience of chronic illness. As Frank

31. Ibid., 13.
32. Frank, *The Wounded Storyteller*, 98.
33. Stahl, "Living into My Image," 2–3.

notes, restitution is about the triumph of biomedicine, while chaos is about suffering so great that the story falters and flounders.[34]

The third type he describes is the quest narrative: "defined by the ill person's belief that something is to be gained through the experience."[35] Critical to the structure of the quest story is that the teller *has* a story to tell—there is both structure and meaning. Common to many quest narratives, the storyteller employs the trope of a journey and takes a reflexive position; Stahl is no exception. In the penultimate portion of her story, "Living in Art," she writes of gaining distance and reflecting intentionally on her "ventures in the world of medicine." Even more illustrative of the quest narrative is its facet of automythology, the rebirth or reinvention of the self because of illness experience. For Stahl, this process begins when, alongside her sister, she newly perceives the images of her body produced by medical imaging technology. It continues toward both an aesthetic appreciation and ultimate reclamation of her body from "the power of medicine" and "its objectifying gaze." And it concludes with an evocation of the Phoenix, the metaphor most dominant in quest stories: "I see myself becoming something new."[36]

ON IDENTITY

> To view your life as blessed does not require you to deny your pain. It simply demands a more complicated vision, one in which a condition or event is not either good or bad but is, rather, both good and bad . . . . In my experience, the more such ambivalences you can hold in your head, the better off you are.[37]

Turner is emphatic that liminality be understood as transformation—a change in being rather than a mere acquisition of

34. Frank, *The Wounded Storyteller*, 115.
35. Ibid.
36. Stahl, "Living into My Image," 19.
37. Mairs, *Carnal Acts: Essays*, 15.

knowledge.[38] To illustrate the experience of the sudden and un-expected passage from a state of health to a state of illness, Frank cites Ronald Dworkin's description of "narrative wreckage," which requires one to weather the storm, map a new course, and steer a different path.[39] Stories such as Stahl's often expose beliefs about temporality: that a past leads naturally into a present that sets up a future.[40] For example, barely launched into adulthood, Stahl links up a series of recognitions and events—the decision to attend divinity school, the dream of ordination, the hope of changing the world—that reflect her (and our own) naïve expectation of a stable relation between what happens in the present and what will happen in the future. Until, she writes, "my feet went numb and the fun stopped."[41] Illness fractures the temporal structure of the life narrative; it obscures the view and demands a detour.

Little et al. point out that when the structures of our lives are suddenly made visible by a diagnosis of serious or chronic disease, "we confront the fear of dying, of pain, of decline and degradation," which is a part of the experience of liminality.[42] Narrative can not only give voice and validate the intermediate position between sickness and health but can also make claims about identity, revealing both a self that is lost and found through the experience. Stahl's epiphany comes when the images that once conveyed fragmentation and dissolution of a single self now represent the multiplicity and possibility of different selves: "This image was of me, but one that was hard to reconcile with the image of myself I am accustomed to seeing in the mirror. After my initial shock, I began to appreciate how the images captured various parts of my body and evoked multiple aspects of my self-understanding."[43]

By inviting others to scan and interpret her story as text *and* as image, Stahl traverses that third phase of the rites of passage,

38. Turner, *The Ritual Process*, 95.
39. Frank, *The Wounded Storyteller*, 54.
40. Ibid., 55.
41. Stahl, "Living into My Image," 4.
42. Little et al. "Liminality," 1491.
43. Stahl, "Living into My Image," 18.

transformation, in which knowledge and wisdom are not simply an aggregation of words and sentences but have ontological value—they re-make the very being of the person. Such a transformation is most vividly expressed in Stahl's awareness, acceptance, and even celebration of the body's complexity, irreducibility, and ambiguity; she is now able and willing to do what Nancy Mairs suggests—hold all such ambivalences in her head. Despite what has happened or might happen, the purpose of the story is now hers to determine: "I no longer strive to acquire a stable body or identity; instead, I have come to value the becoming and unfolding of life . . . ."[44]

BIBLIOGRAPHY

Charmasz, Kathy. "Stories and Silences: Disclosures and Self in Chronic Illness." *Qualitative Inquiry* 8 (2002) 303–28.

Frank, Arthur W. "Health Stories as Connectors and Subjectifiers." *Health: An Interdisciplinary Journal for the Social Study of Health, Illness and Medicine* 10 (2006) 421–40.

Frankenberg, Ronald. "Sickness as a Cultural Performance: Drama, Trajectory, and Pilgrimage: Root Metaphors and the Making of Social Disease." *International Journal of Health Services* 14 (1986) 603–26.

———. "Stories of Illness as Care of the Self: A Foucauldian Dialogue." *Health: An Interdisciplinary Journal for the Social Study of Health, Illness and Medicine* 2 (1998) 329–48.

———. *The Wounded Storyteller: Body, Illness, and Ethics.* Chicago: University of Chicago Press, 1995.

Grytten, Nina, and Per Maseide. "'When I am together with them I feel more ill': The Stigma of Multiple Sclerosis Experienced in Social Relationships." *Chronic Illness* 2 (2006) 195–208.

Kleinman, Arthur. *The Illness Narratives: Suffering, Healing and the Human Condition.* New York: Basic, 1998.

Leder, Drew. *The Absent Body.* Chicago: University of Chicago Press, 1990.

Little, Miles, et al. "Liminality: A Major Category of the Experience of Cancer Illness." *Social Science and Medicine* 47 (1998) 1485–94.

Mairs, Nancy. *Carnal Acts: Essays.* Boston: Beacon, 1996.

Mattingly, Cheryl. *The Paradox of Hope: Journeys through a Clinical Borderland.* Berkeley: University of California Press, 2010.

Mendelson, Cindy. "Diagnosis: A Liminal State for Women Living with Lupus." *Health Care for Women International* 30 (2009) 390–407.

44. Ibid., 13.

Turner, Victor. *The Forest of Symbols: Aspects of Ndembu Ritual.* Ithaca, NY: Cornell University Press, 1967.

———. *From Ritual to Theatre: The Human Seriousness of Play.* New York: PAJ, 1982.

———. *The Ritual Process: Structure and Anti-Structure.* Chicago: Aldine, 1969.

Van Gennep, Arnold. *The Rites of Passage.* Chicago: University of Chicago Press, 1961.

4

TechnoVision

Seeing through the Scanner

KIRSTEN OSTHERR

INTRODUCTION

Ever since the discovery of X-rays gave us the capacity to see inside of a living human body without cutting it open, medical ways of seeing the body have been technologically mediated.[1] In recent decades, the increasing biomedicalization of daily life has led to a rapid expansion of practices for technological mediation of the body.[2] In this context, medical imaging has been enshrined as the paramount arbiter of health and disease, subordinating all other forms of knowing. The seemingly objective renderings of human pathology that are presented through scientific technologies

1. On the transformative effect of the X-ray, see Howell, *Technology in the Hospital.*

2. Clarke et al., *Biomedicalization.*

of representation are often sought by doctors and patients as concrete, visible clues to hidden forms of suffering. Yet, for patients, the affirmation of objective truth is rarely the primary experience that emerges from encounters with imaging studies of their own bodies. This chapter will explore the tension between the subjective experience of pain and illness and the technologies of medical visualization that claim to document and define those experiences through practices of measurement and quantification.

Emerging at the blurry intersection of personal and scientific representation is the artistic rendering of the patient's experience. This chapter will begin by situating Devan Stahl's imaging studies within the history of medical technovision, asking how the experience of being a patient changes when new imaging technologies show us new dimensions of the human body. Moving from the language of objectivity associated with scientific representation to the language of subjectivity associated with artistic representation, the chapter will discuss the art works based on the imaging studies in the context of patient empowerment movements. By exploring the ways that patients have recently used creative forms of expression to claim ownership of their own data and bodies, the second part of this essay will illuminate the complex role of visual imaging in shaping the patient's experience of subjection and resistance to medical power in the twenty-first century. The final section will discuss Darian Goldin Stahl's artistic renderings of the Magnetic Resonance images themselves, in relation to Devan Stahl's narrative representations of the technological experience of medicine in chapter 1 of this book.

IMAGING TECHNOLOGIES AND THE PATIENT EXPERIENCE

"My diagnosis began with an image and now I am left wondering how I should see myself. Chronic illness now shapes my identity, but it leaves no visible scars."[3]

3. Stahl, "Living into My Image," 20, in this volume.

Like "the body multiple" described by Dutch scholar Annemarie Mol, medical visualizations have always lived multiple lives.[4] They exist in the imagination of a culture, through literary and artistic fictions, long before they are ever actualized in the form of hardware. They always aspire to show more than they truly can show. And they always leave doctors and patients wanting more. Medical visualizations also always give us more than we bargained for, showing us things we wish we hadn't seen, things we misunderstand, and things we don't believe. Even though they require interpretation, medical visualizations also serve to halt interpretation, providing a conclusive diagnosis where before there was only a hypothesis, or a worry.[5] Medical images confirm our belief in what is already present but invisible to the naked eye, and they establish the plausibility of other things, as yet unseen. By building self-affirming worlds that shape subsequent medical interventions, imaging technologies integrate creative and empirical data, leading us to see the human body in previously unimaginable ways. For the patient whose body provides the raw material for the imaging study, the boundaries between clinical and fictional images suddenly appear much more permeable than they had previously seemed.

HISTORICAL CONTEXT

The desire to see inside of a living human body, to understand how external manifestations connect to internal phenomena, has a history as old as the historical record. From the early anatomical illustrations of Vesalius's *De humani corporis fabrica* (1543) to the mid-nineteenth-century publication of *Gray's Anatomy: Descriptive and Surgical Theory* (1858), the development of improved techniques of medical visualization has often been driven by a combined need for educational and diagnostic tools. All of the now-familiar modern technologies—from the X-ray through

4. Mol, *The Body Multiple*.
5. See Joyce, *Magnetic Appeal*.

ultrasound, MRI, PET, CT, functional magnetic resonance imaging (fMRI), and high definition fiber tracking (HDFT) scans—have profoundly altered the ways physicians practice medicine, resulting in major advances in the ability to diagnose disease and fewer but substantial advances in treatment as well.[6] The grand federal BRAIN Initiative, announced in 2015, aims to "produce a revolutionary new dynamic picture of the brain that, for the first time, shows how individual cells and complex neural circuits interact in both time and space."[7] The goal of this undertaking is to create a new kind of image that will enable new forms of research and discovery in neuroscience, ultimately translating to disease prevention and improved patient health. However, the exact mechanism for moving from the image to the outcome is less clear; it is based on a belief in the inherent value of novel forms of medical visualization for increasing scientific understanding. The link between seeing and doing at the lab bench takes a great leap of faith to arrive at the patient's bedside.

Medical imaging technologies are continuously developed through an iterative process linking national and international research priorities to new funding mechanisms that facilitate development of novel imaging prototypes that lead to experimentation, commercialization, further refinement of the technology, and always, pursuit of the next thing we wish we could see but cannot. The substantial investment in the ongoing development of novel imaging devices is legitimated through reference to the human beings who will benefit from the advancement of medical science. Yet the true end user—ultimately the patient, not the doctor or technician—is rarely a priority for design specification. Consider Devan Stahl's extended description of her experience inside the MRI scanner, succinctly captured in one memorable phrase, "I never knew I had claustrophobia until I began receiving regular

6. For a technical explanation of how imaging technologies work, see Wolbarst, *Looking Within*. See also Schoonover, *Portraits of the Mind*.

7. U.S. Dept. of Health and Human Services, "What is the BRAIN Initiative?"

MRI exams."[8] No one would describe the experience inside of the MRI scanner as user-centered, but few would dispute the value of the images that result, especially compared to no images at all. In a similar vein, few women would describe the experience of breast mammography as pleasant or even painless. But, at least in the early years of mammography, the discomfort was seen as a life-saving compromise, well worth the trouble. In recent years, some debate has emerged regarding the cost-to-benefit ratio and the predictive accuracy of these imaging technologies.[9] Moreover, questions have emerged about who gets imaged and who does not, and what kinds of disparities might result from uneven access to medical imaging. Some studies have questioned the role of racial bias in determining which pediatric patients presenting at the Emergency Department for head trauma will receive a CT scan.[10] While the details of these studies are beyond the scope of this chapter, their broad implications are not. When we look at the entire ecosystem of medical imaging, we discover that the quest to see more, look deeper, and find new things coexists with deep skepticism and doubt about whether these visualizations truly show us more, enable better care, and are worth the cost.[11]

Why, then, do we continue the quest? Perhaps the answer lies in the imaginative draw that novel imaging devices exert on our creative impulses. As media headlines from the discovery of X-rays to the announcement of the BRAIN Initiative demonstrate, these technologies generate a great deal of public interest. The attraction is further evidenced by the multitude of exhibits on medical imaging at museums of science and by their coverage in the popular press, a tradition that scholar Oliver Gaycken has traced back to the nineteenth century.[12] Indeed, the public and

---

8. Devan Stahl, "Living into My Image," 1.

9. Nelson et al. "Harms of Breast Cancer Screening," 256–67 See also Healy et al. "Use of Positron Emission Tomography to Detect Recurrence and Associations with Survival in Patients with Lung and Esophageal Cancer," 1–8.

10. Mannix et al. "Neuroimaging for Pediatric Head Trauma," 694–700.

11. Van Dijck, *The Transparent Body*.

12. Gaycken, *Devices of Curiosity*.

professional interest in expanding the capabilities of medical imaging, especially as a means toward minimally invasive medicine, has sometimes allowed new devices to drive medical practice before their benefits have been proven.[13]

The cultural life of medical imaging clearly plays a role in shaping modes of perception and representation that move between medical science, art, commerce, and popular culture. These blurry boundaries might prompt us to consider how we perceive the division between scientific and artistic techniques of visualization, and why we attribute different values to images depending on where and why they are created. Images produced in a clinical setting tend to be treated as carrying objective, scientific data, while art objects are usually understood as providing subjective, aesthetic renderings of experience. And yet, the very appearance of medical imaging outside of the clinic makes it difficult to define clear boundaries between objective and subjective, science and art, data and experience, even when the observational setting provides strong interpretive cues. Indeed, viewing Devan Stahl's MRI scans in an art gallery produces a profoundly different experience than viewing them in a hospital, even if the same technology is involved in producing both sets of images.

In his work on the early uses of X-rays in medicine, Bernike Pasveer has shown how meaning emerges out of an iterative process of interpretation that moves between the imaging technology, the patient, and the doctor:

> First comes the elaborate, skillful work of encoding medical images in terms of historically specific mediations. Second comes a new body, a body that has the potential of carrying with it phenomena that can be rendered visible through specific technological mediations. In order to refer back to a body, that body too is being loaded with these historical and contemporary characteristics. An image can only signify when it has been transformed

13. See Hillman and Goldsmith, *The Sorcerer's Apprentice.*

by what it refers to, and when what it refers to has been transformed by the imaging technology.[14]

Technologies of visualization from the photograph to the MRI scan are embedded in a complex network of meaning production that shapes them as well as the bodies they image.[15] By examining the different sites and processes of visual representation in medicine, from the imaging center to the art space, we can expand our understanding of how medical ways of seeing work, enabling doctors and patients to perceive health and disease, imagine possible treatments, and visualize future cures.

PATIENT EMPOWERMENT THROUGH (SOCIAL USES OF) TECHNOLOGY

The first part of this chapter framed Devan Stahl and Darian Goldin Stahl's collaborative artwork through the history of medical imaging technologies, emphasizing the role of interpretation within and beyond the clinical context as a space for opening up alternative forms of visual knowledge. This section will expand on that concept by exploring another key facet of the technomediated patient experience in the twenty-first century: the "democratization" of access to information and communication technologies, and the emergence of new platforms for patient expression that arose as a result.

Devan Stahl's effort to reclaim her self-identity by asserting her own interpretation of her medical images alongside a trusted collaborator may have grown out of a private process of reflection and discovery. But through this work, Stahl participates in a growing public movement, sometimes called the "e-patient" movement, which offers an important frame for understanding how medical power hierarchies are shifting in response to patient activism. A central feature of this movement for our present focus is the role of

14. Pasveer, "Representing or Mediating," in Pauwels, *Visual Cultures of Science*, 59.

15. Dumit, *Picturing Personhood*; Saunders, *CT Suite*.

expressive media, including visual art, creative writing, and video that can spread through the social networks of the mobile web to engage and empower voices that had formerly been silenced.

The term "e-patient" was defined by Dr. Tom Ferguson and the e-patient working group as "individuals who are equipped, enabled, empowered and engaged in their health and health care decisions."[16] A key facilitator of all of these "e's" is the "e" of "email" and "e-health," which refers in this case to the internet and the worldwide web more broadly, as sources of information and platforms for connection that help foster much of the empowerment and engagement that contemporary e-patients have within their reach. In many ways, this last "e" changed everything. This is the same "e" that played such a powerful role in the social network revolution and the internet revolution that have given rise to social justice movements around the world, from the "Arab Spring" to "Occupy Wall Street" and "Black Lives Matter."[17]

The e-patient movement is central to understanding how the voices of patients like Devan Stahl have grown louder in the digital age, because this movement is focused on using digital tools to create access to information and connection to geographically dispersed communities, for the purpose of meeting healthcare needs. But in order for patients to be optimally engaged in their healthcare, some aspects of the traditional doctor-patient relationship would have to change. For example, the idea that the doctor is the gatekeeper to knowledge is overturned when patients can access information from open resources and from each other online. Similarly, the power to interpret images becomes a matter of creative dispute when artists adapt scientific imaging practices to provide a more subjective rendering of the patient experience. In this way, the whole idea of the e-patient movement is disruptive, because it challenges long-held orthodoxies and power structures in medicine.

16. Ferguson et al. "e-patients: How They Can Help Us Heal Healthcare," ii.

17. Rainie and Wellman, *Networked*; Hussain and Howard, "What Best Explains the Successful Protest Cascades?" 48–66; Schwartz, "Pre-Occupied"; Stephen, "How Black Lives Matter Uses Social Media to Fight the Power."

In fact, e-patients are part of a long history of activism around social justice and healthcare, with important roots in HIV/AIDS activism in the late-1980s and early-1990s. The struggle to control public representations of people with AIDS played a key role in this movement.[18] Mass media actively shaped perceptions about HIV/AIDS, and consequently, they also became a target for activists who felt that information and understanding about AIDS was being shaped by vested interests who did not care enough about the people who were dying from this new disease.[19] In the pre-internet era, most Americans received their news from print media like newspapers and magazines, as well as mass media like television and radio.[20] In this top-down, broadcast model it was difficult for less powerful members of society to have their voices heard. But many of the AIDS activist groups, in particular the AIDS Coalition to Unleash Power (ACT-UP), used a media-savvy civil disobedience strategy to ensure coverage of their protests by mainstream news outlets.[21] By working to take back control over their own images and their own voices in the mass media, AIDS activists accomplished great feats. Seeing the e-patient movement as part of this legacy puts the current movement in a meaningful historical context.

Since the early years of AIDS activism, there has been a real transformation in the ways that patients can connect online and access web resources, and the movement has changed as these tools have evolved. In the early days of the internet, patients were able to use it to access information from read-only files—this was a significant step forward from not having any access to other patients or medical information, but it was only a first step. In the second phase of this movement, the social web enabled the beginnings of peer-to-peer healthcare. As the web matured and expanded

18. Crimp, *AIDS*; Triechler, *How to Have Theory in an Epidemic*.

19. Epstein, *Impure Science*.

20. Hilmes, *Only Connect*.

21. For a rich archive of documentation about the role of ACT-UP in AIDS activism in this era, see the ACT-UP Oral History Project, available at: http://www.actuporalhistory.org.

from being an open repository of information to a site for communication and exchange, patients found each other and formed robust social networks of tremendous value to the participants.[22] Now, in the era of do-it-yourself content creation, e-patients are not just communicating with each other, they're also building databases online, conducting their own scientific experiments, sharing creative output, and helping shape the era of participatory, patient-centered medicine. We've entered the era of peer-to-peer healthcare.[23]

This context matters for our understanding of Devan Stahl and Darian Goldin Stahl's art collaboration, because patient self-expression, regardless of whether it takes place in a born-digital format or an ancient paper-based artistic medium, has been amplified in recent years through social networks that can provide new forms of collective experience. Instead of struggling in isolation, patients like Devan can see themselves as people who are part of a community, part physical, part virtual, that values alternative understandings of medical images and data. Indeed, a significant theme in the e-patient dialogue has centered on access to and ownership of patient data. Patient activist Hugo Campos notably fought a medical device manufacturer for access to his implanted cardiac defibrillator data.[24] Artist Regina Holliday fought several hospitals for access to her dying husband's medical imaging studies, and created "The Walking Gallery" art project to give expression to that struggle.[25] And "e-patient Dave" deBronkart launched the catchphrase "gimme my damn data" to give voice to the collective outrage that patients felt at not being entrusted with the contents of their own medical records.[26] A feeling of ownership over one's own self-image plays an integral role in the formation of

22. Vartabedian, "The Case for New Physician Literacies in the Digital Age."

23. Fox, "Peer-to-Peer Healthcare."

24. Singer, "Getting Health Data from Inside Your Body."

25. Barr, "Activist Ignites a Movement for Patients through Art and Story"; Holliday, "Access to Your Record Can Save Your Life."

26. DeBronkart, "How the ePatient Community Helped Save My Life."

patient empowerment in the e-patient data liberation movement and in the Stahls' work to reclaim the meaning of Devan's MRI scans. As we will see in the next section, Darian's manipulation of the medical imaging studies transforms those visualizations aesthetically, and thereby reframes the power dynamics embedded in the power of the medical gaze.

THE ARTWORKS: SEEING THROUGH THE SCANNER

We will now turn to Devan Stahl's reappropriation of her own MRI scans for use by her sister, the artist Darian Goldin Stahl. As framed by Devan's own writings about her experience of imaging, diagnosis, and participation in a clinical trial for a new multiple sclerosis drug, the artistic renderings of the MRI scans suggest a purposeful act of reclaiming. Devan described her experience of constant, intrusive examinations as she endured "numerous MRIs, echocardiograms, electrocardiograms, pulmonary function tests, eye exams, blood tests, walking tests, dexterity tests, and memory tests," finally realizing, "I was not receiving medical care; I was a guinea pig. I was testing a product."[27] Goldin Stahl did not adapt the imaging studies simply because they were aesthetically interesting source material, though they certainly have served that function. Instead, she adapted the original clinical images because they had positioned Devan as an object of medical investigation, without agency, voice, or power to resist. Darian's adaptation of those images offers a new interpretation that restores some of the power of self-presentation to the figure in the image, while also exploring the instability often felt by those occupying the subjective role of the "patient."

Goldin Stahl's artworks also reflect the heterogeneity of medicine's visual culture, which includes art works that incorporate medical imaging studies as well as art whose aesthetics are inspired by medical technologies of seeing, whether directly or indirectly. Art

27. Stahl, "Living into My Image," 10.

historians have noted the creative inspiration that surrealists, cubists, and other avant-garde artists have gained from X-ray imaging since the late nineteenth century; many have identified Marcel Duchamp's *Nude Descending a Staircase* (1912) as an exemplary artwork influenced by the visual perception of bodily fragmentation produced through X-ray imaging and chronophotography.[28] Indeed, the history of art is full of such examples, continuing in the present through the work of artists such as Goldin Stahl.

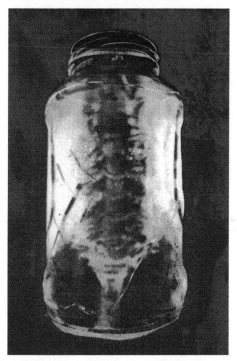

"The Vessel," Silkscreen, 13" x 9," 2013 here

Evocative of the collections of pathological specimens often displayed in medical museums and anatomical theaters of the nineteenth century, "The Vessel" (2013) presents a rendering of a spinal cord, captured in a mason jar. As if preserved in a chemical solution for the future instruction of curious medical students, the

28. Henderson, *The Fourth Dimension and Non-Euclidean Geometry in Modern Art.*

body in this image is reduced to its anatomically interesting features. Stripped of human context, this image is packaged for post-mortem consumption, preserving the vestige of a living being in a state incompatible with life. The sense of mortality and grotesque medical display in "The Vessel" exposes the mood of morbidity and dread that the medical imaging apparatus conjures in the bodies subjected to its rays.

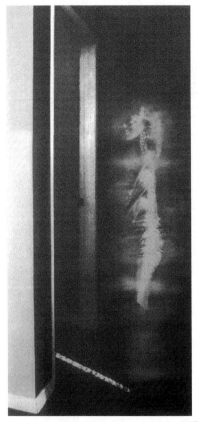

"Hallway," Silkscreen, 84" x 42," 2014 here

In contrast to the feeling of entrapment in "The Vessel," the whole body scan that appears in "Hallway" (2014) conjures a liminal scene of purposeful but evanescent motion toward a threshold of uncertainty. A bright line lights the path forward, and the facial features atop the exposed spinal column blend human with alien imagery, as this figure seems to float across the screen with a determined expression. Operating on an alternate plane of reality, this being sees something that we viewers cannot. It is unclear whether the world beyond the threshold holds promise or threat; for better or worse, the momentum of this figure will not be halted.

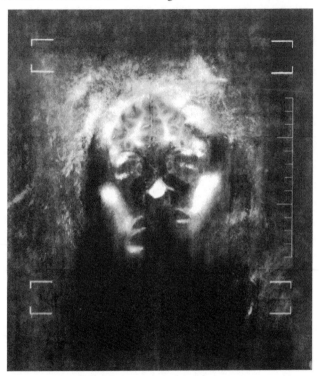

"Becoming Scanned," Lithography and silkscreen, 30" x 28" 2014

The figure in "Becoming Scanned" (2014) seems to be pressing her face against the frame of the imaging viewfinder, struggling to break through. With her face surrounded by a blur of faintly registered hair, the figure seems to emit sparks of agitation from the crown of her head. One hand pressed against the glass emphasizes the sense of entrapment, and the urge to escape. Recalling Devan's commentary on her feelings of claustrophia inside the MRI tunnel, this image brings together the scientific practices of graphing and measuring with the rarely acknowledged emotions that such practices often evoke in their "research subjects." The distinct lack of passivity captured here suggests that this figure will not remain on the "patient" side of the looking glass for long.

CONCLUSION

In our mobile, image-saturated, digitally connected society, the boundaries that have historically divided expert production of medical visualizations from lay consumption of those images have become quite blurry.[29] The ability to produce medical images and display them to patients had formerly rested solely in the hands of physicians, who exercised complete control over a patient's access to those images, which always took place within a formal clinical setting. With our ability to easily move digital images and data in the twenty-first century, these images have escaped the clinic, moving into the hands of activated patients and creative artists alike. The blurring of clinical and artistic images is reflected in novel approaches to visual art, including the Stahls' collaboration.

In the past two decades, visual art has become a central aspect of medical center design, and many hospitals now host evidence-based programs that help patients produce art works as part of their healing process.[30] At the same time, many visual artists working in studios find the human body to be a rich source of imagery. In this context, medical images become art objects that are consumed by patients, physicians, and the general public (most of whom become patients at some point in their lives), in a diversity of settings. For example, in 2009, curators brought together artists from the Orange County Center for Contemporary Art in Santa Ana, California, and imaging specialists from the Mission Hospital in Mission Viejo, California, to produce an art show called *The Art of Imaging*.[31] The exhibit included artworks that manipulated

29. Sturken and Cartwright, *Practices of Looking*.

30. Ulrich, "The Arts of Healing," 1779–81.

31. The Orange County Register, "Medicine, High-tech and Art Unite in Santa Ana."

X-rays and CT scans to produce complex images that foreground-ed the aesthetic qualities inherent in all visual representations, qualities that are often suppressed within the clinical setting. Any of these artistic productions can be easily uploaded to the Internet and shared with vast communities, who might repurpose them in unpredictable ways. In this sense, even the conceptual division between producers and consumers of medical images has broken down, through the shift from an old "read-only" media technology culture to a new digital "read-write" culture.[32] As these images travel outside of the clinic and across the Internet, they acquire new meanings and prompt the formation of unpredictable new alliances.

As part of this movement, the Stahls' collaborative artwork demonstrates the power of reclaiming the technomediated patient narrative, particularly through the use of creative forms of expression. Many patients have experienced the uncanny feeling of seeing their bodies rendered as beautiful yet alien forms in medical imaging studies. The Stahls' project offers a vivid example of how that source material, often acquired under painful circumstances, can nonetheless provide an opportunity for reflection, recuperation of narrative power, and beauty. Medical centers would do well to learn from this model and create opportunities for their patients to engage with the visual artifacts of clinical encounters. Not only would patients benefit from the experience, as Devan Stahl can attest, but clinicians and other healthcare professionals might find valuable new meanings in the reinterpretation of their medical visualizations as well.

BIBLIOGRAPHY

Barr, Sarah. "Activist Ignites a Movement for Patients through Art and Story." *Kaiser Health News* (February 22, 2013). http://khn.org/news/regina-holliday-patient-advocate.

Bijan, Stephen. "How Black Lives Matter Uses Social Media to Fight the Power." *Wired* (November 2015). http://www.wired.com/2015/10/how-black-lives-matter-uses-social-media-to-fight-the-power.

32. Lessig, *Remix.*

Clarke, Adele E., et al., eds. *Biomedicalization: Technoscience, Health, and Illness in the U.S.* Durham, NC: Duke University Press, 2010.

Crimp, Douglas. *AIDS: Cultural Analysis, Cultural Activism.* Cambridge: MIT Press, 1988.

DeBronkart, Dave. "How the ePatient Community Helped Save My Life." *British Medical Journal* 346 (2013) f1990.

Dijck, José van. *The Transparent Body: A Cultural Analysis of Medical Imaging.* Seattle: University of Washington Press, 2005.

Dumit, Joseph. *Picturing Personhood: Brain Scans and Biomedical Identity.* Princeton: Princeton University Press, 2004.

Epstein, Steven. *Impure Science: AIDS, Activism, and the Politics of Knowledge.* Berkeley: University of California Press, 1996.

Ferguson, Tom, with the e-Patients Scholars Working Group. "e-patients: How They Can Help Us Heal Healthcare" (2007). http://e-patients.net.

Fox, Susannah. "Peer-to-Peer Healthcare." Pew Research Center Report (February 28, 2011). http://www.pewinternet.org/2011/02/28/peer-to-peer-health-care-2.

Gaycken, Oliver. *Devices of Curiosity: Early Cinema and Popular Science.* New York: Oxford University Press, 2015.

Healy, Mark A. Huiying Yin, Rishindra M. Reddy, and Sandra L. Wong. "Use of Positron Emission Tomography to Detect Recurrence and Associations with Survival in Patients with Lung and Esophageal Cancers." *Journal of the National Cancer Institute* 108 (2016) djv429.

Henderson, Linda Dalrymple. *The Fourth Dimension and Non-Euclidean Geometry in Modern Art.* 4th ed. Cambridge: MIT Press, 2013.

Hillman, Bruce J., and Jeff C. Goldsmith. *The Sorcerer's Apprentice: How Imaging Is Changing Health Care.* New York: Oxford University Press, 2011.

Hilmes, Michele. *Only Connect: A Cultural History of Broadcasting in the United States.* 4th ed. Boston: Wadsworth, 2014.

Holliday, Regina. "Access to Your Record Can Save Your Life." Health IT Stories. https://www.healthit.gov/profiles/caregiver/access-to-medical-records.

Howell, Joel D. *Technology in the Hospital: Transforming Patient Care in the Early Twentieth Century.* Baltimore, MD: Johns Hopkins University Press, 1995.

Hussain, Muzammil, and Philip Howard. "What Best Explains the Successful Protest Cascades? ICTs and the Fuzzy Causes of the Arab Spring." *International Studies Review* 15 (2013) 48–66.

Joyce, Kelly A. *Magnetic Appeal: MRI and the Myth of Transparency.* Ithaca, NY: Cornell University Press, 2008.

Lessig, Lawrence. *Remix: Making Art and Commerce Thrive in the Hybrid Economy.* New York: Penguin, 2009.

Mannix, Rebekah, et al. "Neuroimaging for Pediatric Head Trauma: Do Patient and Hospital Characteristics Influence Who Gets Imaged?" *Academic Emergency Medicine: Official Journal of the Society for Academic Emergency Medicine* 17 (2010) 694–700.

Mol, Annemarie. *The Body Multiple: Ontology in Medical Practice*. Durham, NC: Duke University Press, 2002.

Nelson, H. D., et al. "Harms of Breast Cancer Screening: Systematic Review to Update the 2009 U.S. Preventive Services Task Force Recommendation." *Annals of Internal Medicine* 164 (2016) 256–67.

The Orange County Register. "Medicine, High-tech and Art Unite in Santa Ana" (February 14, 2009). http://www.ocregister.com/entertainment/art-93316-imaging-hospital.html.

Pauwels, Luc, ed. *Visual Cultures of Science: Rethinking Representational Practices in Knowledge Building and Science Communication*. Lebanon, NH: Dartmouth College Press, 2006.

Rainie, Lee, and Barry Wellman. *Networked: The New Social Operating System*. Cambridge: MIT Press, 2014.

Saunders, Barry. *CT Suite: The Work of Diagnosis in the Age of Noninvasive Cutting*. Durham, NC: Duke University, 2008.

Schoonover, Carl. *Portraits of the Mind: Visualizing the Brain from Antiquity to the 21st Century*. New York: Abrams, 2010.

Schwartz, Mattathias. "Pre-Occupied: The Origins and Future of Occupy Wall Street." *The New Yorker* (November 28, 2011). http://www.newyorker.com/magazine/2011/11/28/pre-occupied.

Singer, Emil. "Getting Health Data from Inside Your Body." *MIT Technology Review* (November 22, 2011). https://www.technologyreview.com/s/426171/getting-health-data-from-inside-your-body.

Sturken, Marita, and Lisa Cartwright. *Practices of Looking: An Introduction to Visual Culture*. 2nd ed. New York: Oxford University Press, 2009.

Triechler, Paula. *How to Have Theory in an Epidemic: Cultural Chronicles of AIDS*. Durham, NC: Duke University Press, 1999.

Ulrich, Roger. "The Arts of Healing." *Journal of the American Medical Association* 281 (1999) 1779–81.

U.S. Dept. of Health and Human Services, National Institutes of Health, The BRAIN Initiative home page. "What is the BRAIN Initiative?" http://www.braininitiative.nih.gov.

Vartabedian, Bryan. "The Case for New Physician Literacies in the Digital Age." 33 charts blog post (September 20, 2012). http://33charts.com/2012/09/new-physician-literacies.html.

Wolbarst, Anthony Brinton. *Looking Within: How X-Ray, CT, MRI, Ultrasound, and Other Medical Images Are Created and How They Help Physicians Save Lives*. Berkeley: University of California Press, 1999.

5

Artful Self-Reflection as Biomedical Intervention
Some Theological Musings

ELLEN T. ARMOUR

The diagnosis began with an image and now I am left wondering how I should see myself.

—Devan Stahl

Technologies of visualization from the photograph to the MRI scan are embedded in a complex network of meaning production that shapes them as well as the bodies they image.

—Kirsten Ostherr

To my knowledge, the volume of which this essay is a part is unique, though not entirely unprecedented. It is a blend of genres, both visual (artwork and MRI scans) and verbal (the scholarly essay, the personal memoir), and of disciplines (visual arts, medical humanities, bioethics, philosophy, theology). I am one of two contributors assigned a distinctive responsibility: to offer reflections on the four essays (and accompanying visual images) that constitute the core of the volume: the memoirs crafted by Devan Stahl and her sister, Darian Goldin Stahl (along with Goldin Stahl's artwork), and the scholarly analyses of their contributions offered by Kirsten Ostherr and Therese Jones. That is no easy task, though I hope to convince you that it is a productive and enlightening one.

Given the mixed nature of this project, I feel compelled to start with the personal before moving to the scholarly register. First, I want to express my gratitude to Devan for inviting me into this singular, brave, and important project. I admire her willingness to share such intimate reflections (in word and image) of and about herself—not only with me and my fellow contributors (whom she knows and chose) but with a wider readership, most of whom she will neither know nor have chosen. My gratitude and admiration, as well, to her sister, Darian, first and foremost for the amazing visual "translations," as she aptly dubs them, of Devan's MRI scans into works of art. They are matched in creativity and insight by the narrative that she provides to accompany her art; one that situates her creative process within the larger sisterly task of coming to terms with Devan's diagnosis. Like Jones and Ostherr, I find both sisters' work profoundly generative. Finally, my gratitude to Jones and Ostherr for their thoughtful and equally generative reflections on Devan's and Darian's work. (N.B. While I will follow scholarly convention and refer to Jones and Ostherr by their last names, I will, with their permission, refer to Devan and Darian by their first names throughout. I do this as a constant reminder to myself, as I write, and my readers, as they read, of their humanity, their singularity, and their intimate connection to one another; dimensions of their contributions—the fundament for the volume—that I hope to honor.)

Second, some words about my own point of entry into this project. My connection to it is both personal and professional. I am, as you know from Devan's introduction, a theologian. In my scholarship and teaching, I work critically and constructively on and with Christian traditions, which I approach through a multi-disciplinary frame formed by theories and theologies of gender, sexuality, race, and by contemporary continental philosophy and, more recently, of postcoloniality, disability, and visual culture theory. Certainly, some of those interests reflect my particular subject position; that is, both how I "identify," as we say these days (as a white, lesbian, able-bodied, cis-gendered feminist), and by my theo-ethical commitments (to social justice and to allyship with non-white, trans, and/or formerly colonized people as well as people living with disabilities). But they also reflect my life experience in a wider way, including my experience with serious illness—which has been, to date, exclusively at second hand. I was Devan's academic advisor at Vanderbilt Divinity School and in that capacity witnessed a (very small) piece of the journey into living openly with MS that she describes herein. I have accompanied dear friends through terminal illness and, am now (along with my brothers) doing something similar (as much as I can from a distance) with my elderly mother and father, who have chronic and progressive illnesses themselves. But it's perhaps my third-hand experience that is distinctive. My spouse is a physical therapist who works primarily with neurologically impaired people; survivors of stroke, various brain cancers, people with chronic and progressive neurological diseases, including MS. Listening to her stories—the happy ones and the heartbreaking ones—has taught me much about the creative possibilities that, though always limited, inhere in us—individually and collectively—even in the face of serious trauma. It has taught me a great deal, as well, about the asymmetrically distributed costs and benefits (emotional as well as financial)—and resulting inequities and cruelties—of our medical system to patients and, in some cases, to providers who truly care for them.

These issues are central to my current scholarship, which is focused on the larger complex relationship between the (modern) self and the systems that produce and sustain it (or not), a relationship in which visual imagery and contemporary biomedicine figure prominently. In my recently published monograph, *Signs and*

Wonders: Theology After Modernity, I take up the vexed question of whether our time and place is rightly described as "postmodern." Modernity may indeed be on its way out, but I resist the notion that we are beyond it arguing instead that we remain beholden to many of its structures and systems; structures and systems that are themselves showing signs of wear and tear. I engage this question through reflections on four sets of photographs and the events they index, all of which took place between 2003 and 2005: the consecration of the Rev. R. Gene Robinson, an openly gay man, to the Anglican episcopacy; two of the photographs from Abu Ghraib; two photographs from Hurricane Katrina; and two video stills of the late Terri Schiavo.

These photographs and the events to which they refer open up and onto crucial challenges that we confront in our time and place; challenges that expose distinctively modern ways of knowing, doing, and being and their limits. I make this case primarily by drawing on the work of the French philosopher and cultural theorist Michel Foucault. Modern knowing, doing, and being are deeply in-formed by (imbricated in, imbued with, shaped by) two distinctive forms of power and knowledge that emerge in modernity, he argues. We typically think of power as domination or control—over oneself or over another. Those who have power are able to exercise their own agency in a given situation; those who don't are subjected to the agency of someone else. This way of thinking about power has its roots in what Foucault calls sovereign power, which has been with us since ancient times. It operates from the top down and takes its crudest, if also emblematic, form in the sovereign's power to kill his subjects.

The distinctively modern forms of power, however, which Foucault dubs biopower and disciplinary power, are more complex in their effects and in their constitution. Channeled through such institutions as families and schools, workplaces and prisons, clinics and asylums, disciplinary power seeks to form individuals into docile subjects—good boys and girls, normal men and women, nurturing mothers and masterful fathers, productive workers and repentant prisoners, and cooperative patients. Both sovereign power and disciplinary power are conscripted into the service of biopower. In lieu of the sovereign's right to kill his subjects, biopower nurtures the lives of certain of its subjects while allowing others to die. In the name of the people, it works on and through the individual (aided and abetted by disciplinary power) but its ultimate targets are populations, its aim the survival and flourishing of the (human) species.

Although Foucault doesn't explicitly thematize this, I see in his work evidence that modern power is channeled through what I call a fourfold made up of "man" (a term Foucault reserves for the modern subject), his raced and sexed others, his divine other, and his animal other. Man occupies the center while his others surround him like a network of mirrors that reflect man back to himself, thus securing his boundaries and his sense of mastery— over himself, over his others, and ultimately over life and death. As modern power's conduit, the fourfold affects how those subjected to that power (that is, thanks to colonialism and its heir, globalization, all of us) become, live, and die. Of course, power begets resistance; and biopower is no exception. The spread of mechanisms of normalization, Foucault tells us, provoked simultaneously the assertion of demands for freedom from its constraints—waged, significantly, in the name of life. To be specific, in the name of "the 'right' to life" as a right "to one's body, to health, to happiness, to the satisfaction of needs, and beyond all the oppressions or 'alienations,' the 'right' to rediscover what one is and all that one can be."[1] We live out our lives, then—individually and collectively—by conforming to or resisting modern power's normative demands.

These modern forms of power are also forms of knowledge, a fact that is particularly important for what I'll say below. That Foucault speaks of *bio*power reflects signal epistemological shifts in what is known, how it's known, and who knows it that are constitutive of modernity; one that tracks with the emergence of the biological sciences out of natural history. If "nature" was a grid of similarities and differences visible on the surface of things, access to the similarities and differences among (especially living)

1. Foucault, *History of Sexuality,* 145.

things requires going beneath the visible surface and plumbing the depths below (think anatomy and dissection, the X-ray and the MRI). This new way of knowing is also a new way of seeing, then, and one that gave rise to and is embedded in modern forms of visual technology, including but not limited to photography.

Finally, theology is directly implicated in that shift. Before modernity's advent, God was understood to be the ultimate source of both nature and (knowledge of) its history. In modernity, however, man displaces God as the one-who-knows. Man looks into the depths of things in order to determine what makes them tick. Yet to displace is not exactly to replace, as man is not God's equal. Unlike God, man's ability to know is limited by time and space; any particular instance of knowing is contingent on "the spatiality of the body, the yawning of desire, and the time of language," as Foucault puts it.[2] Moreover, as both a type of *bios* himself and the one-who-knows *bios*, man is "a strange empirico-transcendental doublet," Foucault writes, who is both subject to and subject of modern knowing.[3] In the so-called human sciences, for example, modern subjects are the source and site of empirical data, the collectors and analysts of that data, and the creators (and sometimes critics) of the frameworks that guide its collection and analysis.

My reference to the human sciences was deliberate as some of them (physiology, for example) are foundational to the practice of modern biomedicine, which is, in turn, foundational to the self-reflections that constitute *this* project. Bio-disciplinary knowing and seeing—who knows and what they know, who sees and what they see—are integral to the practice of biomedicine and the role that MRI's and other visual technologies play in it. As I'll show below, Devan's account of her interactions with biomedical practice demonstrate this. But Devan and Darian deploy other modes of seeing and knowing that are explicitly intended to resist certain effects of biomedical practice; modes that reflect their own personal and professional commitments and training. As Jones and Ostherr show, although they bring particular skill and knowledge

2. Foucault, *The Order of Things*, 315.

3. Ibid., 318.

to the task, Devan and Darian are not alone in pursuing resistance by these means. My focus, in what follows, will be tracing the interaction between bio-disciplinary seeing and knowing and the alternatives put forward here in pursuit of resistance. I hope, by doing so, to advance the goal of ethical intervention in biomedical practice articulated by all four contributors as the larger purpose of this project.

These interactions take place in both narrative and visual modes. The *ur*-narrative, if you will, is the story Devan relays for us of coming to terms with her diagnosis with multiple sclerosis. Visual imagery is central to that story because medical imaging played such a central role in her diagnosis and in the ongoing process of living with MS. Those images, in turn, anchor Darian's creative visual translations, several of which we encounter embedded in her own narrative of their creation (itself part of her processing of Devan's diagnosis). In creating and sharing their work, Devan and Darian explicitly target aspects of the practice of biomedicine that reduce people with illnesses to little more than objects of their disease and its medical treatment. Jones and Ostherr position Devan's and Darian's work in the context of larger cultural currents of similar responses to biomedicine. Jones considers Devan's narrative as an example of the larger genre of pathography (first person narratives of illness). Ostherr focuses on their collaborative art project, in particular, as an example of the larger "e-patient" movement wherein patients reclaim ownership of their experience of illness, often through artistic expression. Both Jones and Ostherr, then, give us deeper insights into how narrative and visual image can be marshaled—by Devan and Darian and others—to resist the debilitating effects of biomedical objectification. Taken together, Devan, Darian, Jones, and Ostherr give us a much more complex tale of what we need to negotiate the psychological costs and benefits, if you will, of modern biomedicine. Those complexities emerge more clearly, I think, when their work is read with some of the insights from *Signs and Wonders* in mind.

***

Being diagnosed with MS initially provokes something of an identity crisis for Devan, the contours of which she limns quite powerfully for her readers. Biomedicine draws her in initially by holding out the promise of knowing the cause of her perplexing symptoms *and* a cure (or at least a treatment regimen) for them. But accessing those promises requires that Devan submit to biomedical objectification as she is stripped down (literally and figuratively) to nothing but a diseased body. If the mechanisms of diagnosis inaugurate that stripping down, its delivery—given with little if any thought to its impact on the person receiving it—completes it. Much of Devan's narrative, then, is an account of her process of self-reconstruction; of incorporating MS into a new sense of who she is. Biomedicine's role in that process doesn't end with diagnosis, of course. As an MS patient, she needs treatment and monitoring. Accessing those services continues to require from her not only submission to objectification, but various forms of self-subjection. *Living* with MS means an ongoing visceral back-and-forth, push-and-pull with biomedicine—both as a patient and as a (voluntary) "guinea pig," as Devan so aptly puts it, in a clinical trial. She must cede knowledge of *how* she is and thus *who* she is to the experts and their diagnostic tools. She must comply with treatment protocols (including repeated MRI's), find ways to pay her portion of the cost of treatment, and along the way interact with the various agents (mechanical and human) of the biomedical system. And gender is not insignificant (along with race and sexuality) to all of this as Devan (an attractive, young, white, and presumptively straight and cis-gendered woman) finds herself exposed to patronizing or perverse interactions with (male) medical professionals. Her narrative conveys viscerally and powerfully the reductive effects of biomedical objectification and self-subjection, and her laudably stubborn resistance to those effects.

Devan is not the first or the last to go public with her account of living with illness. Indeed, memoirs of living with illness have become their own genre—the pathography, per Jones—complete with subgenres. According to Jones, of the three subgenres of pathography, Devan's fits the third, that of the quest narrative. Devan's pathography starts with a plunge into a liminal state inaugurated by the initial shock of diagnosis. As she moves toward accepting and even embracing her diagnosis, Devan emerges from that liminal space with an identity remade around accepting her illness. This remade identity enables her to reclaim a reformed sense of agency, on Jones' read. While it's certainly the case that Devan's new identity and sense of agency isn't a result of biomedical triumph (it's not a restitution narrative, the genre of pathography we prefer, according to Jones), it's also not a heroic narrative of triumph over biomedicine. It is, rather, a narrative of her complex negotiations with biomedicine. The new Devan is born out of the push-and-pull of objectification, self-subjection, and resistance that is biomedical subjection. Like a pearl that takes shape around a grain of sand, this new Devan comes to be in and around the residual scar tissue created by her diagnosis and the immersion into biomedicine that it inaugurated and continues to require. Her negotiations with biomedical subjection are both verbal and visceral, conscious and unconscious, (hopefully) life sustaining and (troublingly) death dealing.

Darian is motivated to take up the artistic remaking of Devan's MRI scans out of her desire to support her sister's coming to terms with her diagnosis. In particular, she hopes in her work to give visual voice, if you will, to Devan's insistent resistance to the demeaning effects of biomedical subjection. Darian brings to the project many things—not least of which is her remarkably creative and insightful way of seeing. That vision enables her to see (Devan, her scans, shadows on the wall) differently. First and perhaps foremost, her artistic gaze enables her to see *through*—that is, into and beyond—what Foucault calls the medical gaze.[4] A hallmark of the medical gaze in our time, according to Ostherr, is its increasing

4. Foucault, *The Birth of the Clinic*. The concept of an objectifying gaze is not distinct to biomedicine; it has its counterparts in art historical discourses (cf. Laura Mulvey's groundbreaking "Visual Pleasure and Narrative Cinema," on the male gaze) and in disability theory (cf. Rosemarie Garland Thomson's *Staring*).

development of and reliance on "technovision," including the MRI. Like its predecessor, the X-ray, the MRI was developed to better enable physicians to diagnose and treat a larger variety of ailments by allowing them to see into the human body in increasing depth and detail. Tellingly, Ostherr notes, technovisual machines have not been designed with the comfort of the patient in mind; an understatement when it comes to the MRI, given Devan's account of the experience.

Technovisual machines channel biopower as a form not only of seeing but of knowing. In doing so, they also channel biomedical subjection as objectification and self-subjection. Both Darian and Devan report looking in vain, to begin with, in MRI scans for any sign of the person whose body they visually reproduce (in slices and segments, that is). Indeed, the untrained eye can make little sense of MRI scans. Clearly, seeing alone isn't enough; one has to know what to look for and that requires another form of biomedical subjection, (a specific form of) medical training. Yet both eventually come to see through this technovisual medical gaze—thanks in no small part to their collaboration. To that task, both bring different modes of seeing and knowing; a critical eye shaped by her disciplinary training as a biomedical ethicist, in Devan's case; an aesthetic eye shaped by her disciplinary training as an artist. For Darian (and ultimately for Devan), seeing through the technovisual medical gaze also involves a process of incorporation—of the images produced by the MRI into Darian's own creative process and ultimately into the works themselves (in various ways). I say "incorporation" to capture not only the relationship of one form of imagery to another, but to capture as well the tactility and materiality of the work itself. (I am tempted to describe Darian's method as form of transubstantiation, but I digress . . . .) Appropriately, their collaboration culminates in artbooks that, in and through the images materialized in its pages (in Darian's words), "hold [Devan's] narrative, internal anatomy, and skin's surface together for the first time";[5] a result that mirrors in many ways the culmination of Devan's process of incorporation.

5. Goldin Stahl, "Lived Scans," 35, in this volume.

I may lean toward transubstantiation, but Darian uses the metaphor of translation to describe her work's relationship to the MRI scans; an especially apt metaphor given the role that words and numbers play in her creative process and in technovision itself. Decoding and communicating the biomedical knowledge generated by the MRI—even to fellow cognoscenti—requires translating what its images show into words and numbers. Appropriately, both Devan and Darian cite examples of those accompanying texts in their work. The very fact that these translations are needed means that what technovision reveals is contestable, even somewhat ambiguous. In both respects—their reliance on textuality and their inherent ambiguity—MRI's resemble photographs. These days, we take for granted that, absent deliberate alteration, photographs give us unmediated access to a "that-there-then."[6] Yet their truthfulness, if you will, had to be established; a process in which, as I recount in *Signs and Wonders*, bio-disciplinary power (channeled through the fourfold) played an instrumental role. Still, even with photographic truth now rather firmly established, even the most banal photograph does not necessarily immediately convey in full its "that-there-then" to a random viewer. If you haven't seen firsthand that particular object at that particular location at that particular time, you may be left in the dark, as we say. In most cases, information about a photograph's "that-there-then" is conveyed by words. Captions always accompany news media photographs, for example, and we often label our family snapshots. (Indeed, the French philosopher Jacques Rancière, in *Future of the Image*, speaks of visual images as imagetexts; a label that seems apt for MRI scans as well.) And the truth of any given photograph can be disputed. For example, in *Regarding the Pain of Others*, Susan Sontag notes that both sides in the Bosnian civil war used the same photograph (of slaughtered children) to accuse the other of war crimes.

---

6. In using this terminology, I riff off of Roland Barthes' "that-has-been" (*ça-a-été*) in *Camera Lucida*. Barthes' phrase emphasizes photography's relationship to the past at the expense of location and object.

These aspects of visual imagery pertain also to Darian's art-work—both its production and its reception, in my view. Darian makes generative use of the ambivalence built into visual images—whether photographs, MRI's, or the silkscreens she creates—to do these translations. The imagetexts she translates are Devan's MRI scans and their textual accompaniments coupled now with *Devan's* writing about her experiences. But the translations aren't simply from one mode of image to another; they also draw on different visual vocabularies, if you will. While the scans trade exclusively in the medical lexicography, Darian's images work with artistic, medical, and domestic visual lexicons. If the medical lexicon speaks objectivity, the vocabularies with which Darian places it in conversation speak (inter)subjectivity, itself a language of affect as much as object. One more dimension of photographic practice that I discuss in *Signs and Wonders* pertains here. We often speak of how photographs "move" us—emotionally and, in some cases, to take action. (The Abu Ghraib photographs prompted anger and outrage in many viewers, which in turn sparked various forms of protest in the US and abroad, for example.) This affective dimension of visual images is central to the impact and import of Darian's artwork. Central to that is the multidimensionality of Darian and Devan's relationship to each other: they are artist and subject, yes, but also sisters. As I've noted already, Darian appropriately and expertly embeds her description of the process of creating these images in the narrative of her own process of coming-to-terms with Devan's diagnosis—and rightly so, as the artwork she creates is intrinsic to that process. The ways Darian couples the medical and the domestic in her art draws on that multidimensionality. For example, Darian uses her own body as a stand-in for Devan's in many of the images, a strategy that reads to me as an act of sisterly empathy as much as artistic convenience. Viewing those images with Darian's and Devan's narratives in mind amplifies their affective import. "Numb" (2013), for example, features images of Darian's nude body frozen in ice (to suggest the neuropathy that comes with MS, Darian writes). Likewise, "The Vessel" (2013), which features a skeletal image, captured in a jar calls to mind Devan's description of the claustrophobic experience of the MRI tube. But there is yet more, I think. Both "Vessel" and "Numb" call to mind the affective import of dealing with MS. Receiving a life-changing diagnosis—one's own or one's loved one's—can itself invoke an initial numbness as a strategy of self-protection. That reaction will hopefully give way, in due course, to something else. Indeed, the affective dimensions of "Vessel" render that shift legible.

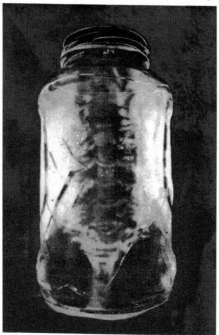

"The Vessel," Silkscreen, 13" x 9," 2013

This image calls to mind the stereotypical childhood experience of catching insects in a jar—only now, of course, with the insect replaced by a human skeleton. The presumptive "innocence" of childhood is replaced by the realities of a present (and an anticipated future) irrevocably shaped for both Devan and her family by progressive chronic illness. The particular mix of the medical (the MRI) and the domestic (the Mason jar that contains it) conveys Devan's transition from family member to patient and the (immediate and anticipated) grief that accompanies it—inflected for me at least, by a touch of nostalgia for a lost childhood. This particular merger of the domestic and the medical both feeds and draws on visual ambivalence. The skeleton invites a medical gaze, which the glass surface of the Mason jar both enables and obscures, thereby humanizing the gaze required to truly see the skeleton the jar contains.

***

However apt readers may find the reflections I have offered so far, they may seem to have strayed a good distance from my main area of expertise, theology. In the space remaining to me, I'll return to my disciplinary home to offer some final reflections. Recall, if you will, that a hallmark of bio-disciplinary power/knowledge is its creation and reliance on man rather than God. As I noted earlier, man displaces God in modernity, but man does not *replace* God. Unlike divine knowing, human knowing is limited by time and space, and yet as the development of biomedicine and the sciences that undergird it make clear, man-the-knower stubbornly and persistently pushes against those limits seeking to know—and control—more and more. And in many ways, man has succeeded. As I note in *Signs and Wonders,* to an unprecedented degree, we now hold the power of life and death in our hands; power that once was understood to belong exclusively to God. Our hold on it is, of course, imperfect as both Hurricane Katrina and the controversy over Terri Schiavo's fate reveal, but it is irrefutable. And we can't wish it away. Indeed, we are in many ways dependent on the goods and services provided by the systems and institutions that bio-disciplinary power/knowledge has built—including biomedicine. At the same time, even biomedicine itself is ambivalent about its propulsion to see and know more. As Ostherr observes, the pursuit of technovision "is based on a belief in the inherent value of novel forms of medical visualization for increasing scientific understanding."[7] However, she continues, "the link between

7. Ostherr, "TechnoVision," 59, in this volume.

seeing and doing at the lab bench takes a great leap of faith to arrive at the patient's bedside. . . . And when we look at the entire
ecosystem of medical imaging, we discover that the quest to see
more, look deeper, and find new things coexists with deep skepticism and doubt about whether these visualizations truly show us
more, enable better care, and are worth the cost."[8]

It is precisely at this place of biomedical ambivalence where
the project Devan and Darian have led us through may intervene
with the greatest effect. The labors of resistance undertaken and
analyzed herein seek a course correction in biomedical practice.
That course correction would result in better—that is, more humane—treatment. (How exactly that would impact biomedicine's
approach to treating the patient's *disease* is a more complicated
question that is beyond the scope of this project.) Pursuing that
goal will require confronting and resisting the bio-disciplinary
theo-logic that underlies so much of the practice of biomedicine:
a theo-logic of mastery over life and death manifest in biomedicine—and in certain forms of resistance to it. Central to e-patient
activism, according to Jones' description, is regaining control over
one's medical records, one's treatment, and ultimately oneself. One
cannot help but hear echoes of Foucault's description of bio-disciplinary resistance made in the name of the right to life.

This, I think, is where anchoring resistance to biomedicine's
dehumanizing effects specifically in the insights that Devan and
Darian together offer is particularly important. Although Devan's
pathography trades, to some degree, in bio-disciplinary resistance,
hers is not a tale of recouped mastery—over herself, her body, or
certainly over her disease (much less over biomedicine). The new
identity and sense of agency that Devan comes to embody is rooted, as Jones notes (quoting Devan), not in a naïve presumption of
bodily stability, but in acceptance of the vicissitudes of bodily becoming. Moreover, Devan did not come to this new place by dint
of her own efforts alone. The collaborative venture she engages in
with Darian is, by her own account, crucial to her coming to see
herself *through* the biomedical gaze differently. And that, in turn

8. Ibid., 60.

(and also by her own account) is key to her coming into her new sense of self.

In the concluding pages of *Signs and Wonders,* I observe that bio-disciplinary power's drive for mastery is rooted in and perpetuates a disavowal of vulnerability. That vulnerability is individual and collective, bodily and social, sensory and affective, verbal and visual. Perhaps a signal contribution of Darian and Devan's collaboration here is the way it acknowledges rather than disavows so many of these dimensions of vulnerability—and, in turn, calls us to do the same. Perhaps this is the fundamental lesson that we, as viewers and readers of their work, can take into our own professional and personal negotiations with biomedicine. Though its reliance on technovisual machines obscures that fact, the practice of biomedicine is at bottom deeply human, like the theo-logic that undergirds it. Its foibles and failures as well as its successes remind us of this every day. Negotiating with this all-too-human system will require collaboration and innovation. It will require cultivating practices of seeing and knowing that, like those modeled here, enable us to see *through* the (bio)medical gaze and the system it supports to a more humane future—for ourselves and, we can hope, for it as well.

BIBLIOGRAPHY

Armour, Ellen T. *Signs and Wonders: Theology After Modernity.* New York: Columbia University Press, 2016.

Barthes, Roland. *Camera Lucida: Reflections on Photography.* New York: Hill and Wang, 1981.

Foucault, Michel. *The Birth of the Clinic: An Archaeology of Medical Perception.* Translated by A. M. Sheridan. New York: Routledge, 1989.

———. *The History of Sexuality, Vol. 1: An Introduction.* Translated by Robert Hurley. New York: Random House, 1978.

———. *The Order of Things: An Archaeology of the Human Sciences.* New York: Vintage, 1994.

Garland Thomson, Rosemarie. *Staring: How We Look.* New York: Oxford University Press, 2009.

Mulvey, Laura. "Visual Pleasure and Narrative Cinema." In *Film Theory and Criticism: Introductory Readings,* edited by Leo Braudy and Marshall Cohen, 833–44. New York: Oxford University Press, 1999.

6

Icons of the Body, Darker Gifts of the Flesh

Jeffrey P. Bishop

I have been given many gifts in my life. Some are mere tokens; others carry a deeper significance. Most gifts that have been given have been forgotten, or have receded into the abyss on which memory rides. Some gifts are very touching; they go too deep to share. Most gifts are given with some expectation of a return, even if only a thank you, or gratitude. Others keep re-giving themselves, reminding one to give thanks. One gift that keeps re-giving itself, or re-gifting itself, hangs on the wall of my office. It was given me by a former graduate student, with gratitude for our time together. It is one of my most prized possessions, if I can be said to possess it.

This gift is a framed print of a piece of art made by my graduate student's sister. It is a composite image. The print is called, "The Scan and the Mirror," and has already been seen in this volume. It is, in part, an image of my graduate student's brain; a representation of her body. It has no resemblance to her body in any way that is easily discernible. There is a face in the image, but it is not her face. Yet it carries so much of who she is, and not merely because it is an image of her brain. It captures a part of her life that she has shared with me from the very beginning of our relationship. It carries with it the frailty of her body. The image is also an image not of her own body alone. It is a composite image of her brain and her sister's face. So the face seen in the print is not that of my graduate student. Her sister gave her own face, her own image, to the print, giving the image a new layer of meaning. Still, to my eye, when I look up to ponder the print, I see only my graduate student. After all, the flesh she shares with her sister is closer to her own flesh, than the flesh she shares with her parents.

Every day when I go into my office, it is there. It reminds me of the first day I met Devan Stahl. She was in her second year of divinity school at Vanderbilt University. A friend and colleague in the divinity school, Ellen Armour (the author of the other commentary in this volume), had put Devan in touch with me. Devan thought she might have an interest in pursuing doctoral work, perhaps in bioethics. As I reflect on our first meeting, it seems that the young woman I met that day was nothing like the person I now know. She seemed preoccupied, and a little awkward. I could not figure out why she seemed so ill at ease. After a few awkward minutes of superficial questions and answers about academics generally, and academic bioethics specifically, our conversation turned to disability. Immediately, Devan became more animated and engaged. She was like a different person, and much more like the person I now know.

After about forty-five minutes, we seemed to have wrapped up all the items that Devan wanted to cover and we began exchanging the requisite niceties of a goodbye. As I was about to rise out of my chair, I asked, "Why do you have such an interest in disability?" I remember her response. It was a fully embodied response. Her eyes widened; she took a sharp, quick, but deep breath, held it for what seemed like several seconds. It was clear that her mind was at work pondering what to say, and how to say it. She sat up more straight in her chair as if to steady herself, as if to gather her strength to withstand a burden. The burden that had preoccupied her mind appeared there in her flesh—in her body, on her face, and in her eyes. It then appeared on her lips as she said, "I have multiple sclerosis." And for the first time, I saw her. Right there, in that moment, the frailty of her flesh, which had preoccupied her mind, appeared clearly in her body. And in her vulnerability, Devan gave me the first of many gifts. She gave me the gift of the vulnerability of her flesh. She would go on to give me the gift of her intelligence in the classroom, and her wit. She blessed me again in giving me that print; and now she gives another gift to me again in her invitation for me to be a respondent in this volume.

I take this volume to be an icon of what it means to be human. By icon, I mean something along the lines of what Jean-Luc Marion means in *God without Being*, namely that the being of the one whose image is represented in pigment shines through the image, transforming, nay constituting the being of the one who stands before the icon. Idols, Marion claims, are creations of the observer, the one who gazes upon the object, the one who foists his propositional truths upon the object. The directionality of intention of the idol is the opposite of the icon.

It seems to me that this directionality of intention—this distinction between idols and icons—is not only true of objects. We can turn the gaze onto ourselves. When one turns the gaze onto the self, one creates what Michel Foucault calls an empirico-transcendental doublet, a sovereign subject, an oxymoron. The one who gazes upon her- or himself, creates an idol of the self, a being that both rules over (thus, it is sovereign) and is subjected to that rule (thus, the subject of the sovereign). While Foucault was interested in aesthetic and ethical self-creation, at the end of his life he gave a series of lectures published as a *The Hermeneutics of the Subject*, in which he claims that before one can follow the oracle at Delphi's command to "know thyself," one must take pains with oneself, to care for the self; and to care for the self, one needs companions, others to co-create oneself. I shall argue in this essay three points, two critical, and one constructive.

The first, critical point is that medicine—indeed much of Western culture—is committed to a power ontology, focusing on the efficacious control of the function of the body at the expense of the meaning and purpose of the body. In relation to subjects and objects, subjects deploy a gaze upon objects, and constitute those objects. When those objects are persons, the result is that the person-objects can suffer under the burden of the gaze of the subject. This is essentially Foucault's critique of the clinic.[1] At times, patients desire physicians to deploy that gaze. At other times, the burden of that gaze can be too much.

The second, critical point that I shall argue is that much of the popular response of patient empowerment literature, including the entire narrative medicine movement, unwittingly feeds into the power ontology at work in Western culture, where the self comes to narrate itself, to create itself, to overcome and take charge of the situation. Few people will quibble with the first critique; many will quibble with the second critique. I feel I must beg forgiveness of my colleagues Kirsten Ostherr and Therese Jones for this critique. I shall strive to be gentle.

The third, and hopefully constructive point is that we are not sovereign-subjects, self-creators, self-narrators at all. Self-creators only produce the solipsistic self, the empirico-transcendental doublet. Rather, we are given our being by others. Were we not given our flesh by others, whom we knew not? Were we not given our mother's very flesh to consume, though we knew it not? Were we not given education, such that we could come to know? There is another gift given us, dare I say it. Is the frailty of flesh not a given?

Can it be a gift—even if a darker gift? After all, all of being comes with its frailties—the darker gifts of being. Perhaps when one sets aside the gaze of self-constitution and permits oneself to be constituted by the other, one is given the fullness of one's being. In giving her being to others, she is given her being back. In submitting herself to Darian, Devan is made whole. In pouring her own being, her own flesh into the art, Darian gives Devan a new creation. In giving that art to the world, it becomes an icon for others. In giving us this book, Devan once again gives herself

---

1. Foucault, *The Birth of the Clinic*.

in all her frailty; she gives herself once again to us. And I, for one, am the richer.

THE FAILING POWERS OF THE FLESH

When flesh comes to mind, it is rarely perceived as a gift. The frailty of flesh is certainly a given. Of course, flesh is always there as a given, a kind of condition for the possibility for anything to come to mind; we do, after all, only come to know the world through the material of the body, through the flesh. Yet, the flesh rarely occupies the mind as an object. In fact, it seems to only come to mind when it is problematic, as Kay Toombs noted years ago and as Havi Carel has recently, and so eloquently, reminded us.[2] Only when one cannot do the things that one hopes to do, only when the pain of the flesh or the limits of the flesh captures the attention does one pay any attention to the body. Only when one thinks one is too fat, or too ugly does it come to mind. Only when it is not what we want it to be, or does not do what we hope it will do, only when it is broken does it become an object of our reflection, an object of our mind. The flesh seems to be a dark gift.

Surely, someone will immediately object to the idea that the flesh only occupies the mind when it is broken. Do we not bathe the body, daily? Do we not feed it; do we not do things to preserve its health? Of course; yes, the body can be seen as an object in the everydayness of life. It is a preoccupation of all embodied living. But then it is a *preoccupation*, something that stands in the background, prior to our desires and projects, hidden, almost forgotten. The care of the body is ordered to something else, to our hopes and projects and purposes; but the body seems almost forgotten in the thrall of its perceived purpose. We might call this phenomenon, the forgetfulness of the body. Yet in its being forgotten, and in its givenness, it becomes the instrument through which the entire world comes to mind, and through which we build our entire world. We might say, as Kay Toombs points out riffing on

2. See Toombs, *The Meaning of Illness*; See also Carel, *Illness*.

Heidegger, that the body is *zuhanden*, ready to hand; it is that in and through which we come to perceive and act on the world. It is a kind of tool, the being of which slips into the background of the attention and intention. And when it is broken, it is manifest as *vorhanden*, present at hand, something like a broken tool, a decontextualized object, foreign, unrecognized, other to the self, almost lifeless.[3]

Devan Stahl describes this feeling, or lack of it, when her flesh came to mind. She writes that, "Then my feet went numb and the fun stopped. A sort of tingling sensation began at my feet and started to slowly creep up my legs. It almost felt as if my feet were mildly asleep, but the tingling lasted for days."[4] Note two things: 1) The lack of sensation, the absence of perception turned her mind to her body, in this case her feet and legs. The body—the feet and legs—are brought to mind, are brought to the foreground, a place where the body is not so comfortable being. 2) Yet, even there at the foreground, the body takes up the secondary position, for what concerned Stahl is that "the fun stopped." Put differently, the body came to mind precisely because her projects—in this case, the project of "an awkward twenty-two-year-old"—were called into question. Devan would have to ask herself, "What is her body for?" and reconfigure the answer that she had presumed in the early part of her life.

"What's a body for?" is a question that sounds odd to the ears of the physician. There is an old "pimp" question that medical students are asked by their professors. A "pimp" question is a question designed to trick medical students, a way of putting them in their place. The question is: "What is the purpose of the heart?" The medical student unwittingly answers, "To pump blood." "No!" the professor answers, "The heart has no purpose. It only has a function. Its function is to pump blood." Devan's neurologist knew the difference between function and purpose. The dissatisfaction that Devan felt with her initial neurologist results from the fact that the

3. Toombs, *The Meaning of Illness*; Heidegger, *Being and Time*, 5–6; 396–401.

4. Stahl, "Living into My Image," 4, in this volume.

purpose of Devan's body cannot be separated from the function of Devan's body, not for Devan. The dualism of function and purpose produced by medical thinking is the source of much disillusionment by patients with medicine. Medicine remains dualistic, not because of some Christian view of the body, as Eric Cassell suggests, but because the function of the body has been severed from the purposes of the body by the scientific endeavor.[5] That was at work in Devan's diagnostician.

I have in several other places argued that, in modern medicine, the body can have no purpose, no final cause to use Aristotelian language.[6] Let's apply this interpretive frame to the first neurologist in Stahl's narrative. There is another saying in medicine: "We see what we look for; we look for what we know." The neurologist looks, not at Stahl's body, but at an image of her body. There he finds a disruption in her body, seen indirectly through the medium of the MRI. He is concerned with Stahl's functional body, not Devan's purposive body. He seems unconcerned that Devan is unable to make sense of what she thought her purpose in life might be. Devan conceived herself as a minister, mother, a person whose future, whose projects assumed a body that functions properly. Even in Devan's own self-conception, the normally functioning body is a necessary condition for the possibility of Devan's self-conception and her own understanding of her future projects.

The doctor, unaware of and even oblivious to Devan's bodily self-conception—her self-understanding of her own projects and purposes—only focuses on the functioning body, not the purposive body. In fact, the doctor's self-conception—of himself as a doctor—would be disrupted and made more complicated if he gets too caught-up in Devan's bodily self-conception. It will only distract him from his goal, namely to restore the material function of her body. For that, he needs only the images of the body, the image that tells him the truth, because he knows what to look for, about

5. Cassell, *The Nature of Suffering and the Goals of Medicine*.

6. See Bishop, "Transhumanism, Metaphysics, and the Posthuman God"; Bishop, *The Anticipatory Corpse*; Bishop, "From Anticipatory Corpse to Posthuman God," 679–95.

Devan's flesh. Her flesh no longer functions properly. He can see that. It seems not to matter to him that Devan has been alienated from her body, that Devan's self-conception has been ruptured; nor, it seems, does it matter to him that her projects and purposes for her life are beginning to seem improbable if not starkly impossible. Put into Marion's language, the MRI of Devan's body became an idol. The gaze of the neurologist happens upon a truth—and all idols speak to some truth, though not the whole truth—of Stahl's dysfunctional body. Devan's purposive body was being set aside, perhaps even sacrificed to the neurologist's idol. No doubt, he was almost oblivious to this sacrifice that he asked of Devan.

This focus on function does not mean that the meaning of Devan's body for Devan, and the purpose for her body ordered to her own larger projects, is of no concern to the doctor. In fact, if you asked him, he would tell you that he hopes to restore the possibility of meaning and purpose for Devan, even while he could not give her any sense of how she understood the meaning and purpose of her body. In fact, he would say that by focusing solely on the function of her body, he hopes to return it to its proper functioning—or least to stave off any further detriment to functioning—so that Devan can continue to live out her life through her body. In short, the neurologist, and most doctors, focus on the function and not the meaning or purpose of the body, because they know that it will decay, that entropy will finally triumph over all bodies. Thus, medicine is committed to a power ontology; that is to say, that medicine holds that power is the fundamental unit of analysis beyond which there can be no other analysis. Entropy and decay—disease, sickness, and illness—are a failure of power. For doctors, it is their purpose to stop entropy, to stave it off as long as they can, which brings us to one final reason why the neurologist does not get caught up in Devan's purposes. If he does stave off entropy, the ultimate failure of the medical enterprise becomes all the more painful for him. If he fails in returning the body to proper functioning, and if he comes to appreciate and love the person, then he will be in a position to mourn the loss of meaning and purpose for Devan. In having kept meaning and purpose at arm's length, leaving Devan alone to ponder the meaning of her failing body, and the loss of purpose that comes with it, he does not have to feel it in the depths of his own being. He can remain impersonal; he can protect himself.

So much dissatisfaction with medicine originates here, where bodily function intersects with purpose and meaning. The medical doctor is confronted with loss of function, but the patient is presented with both the loss of function and the loss of purpose and meaning. The doctor focuses all his energy on the functionality of the body; he will treat the body as a mere object, furthering the alienation that the patient feels from her own body. The source of so much of the dissatisfaction of patients with medicine generally and doctors in particular arises from the divorce of function from purpose and meaning. The patient is left alone with her body, which she thought was for one thing, but turns out to be for another. And she is left alone to figure out whether it can have another purpose or meaning.

THE POWERS OF NARRATIVE

Given that medicine is metaphysically agnostic about any meaning of and purpose for any particular body, we find medicine to be woefully lacking, adding insult to the injury of the loss of meaning and purpose that accompanies failing function. In many ways, the medical humanities buy into this power ontology, by claiming that it is through the power of story that one gains power over one's disease, illness, or sickness.[7] If the body cannot be sewn together such that function can be restored, then we can turn to the medical humanists who will give the possibility of recreating meaning and purpose for the now-scarred body. Put differently, these patient empowerment movements, whether through the e-patient movement or the pathography movement, act as subjectifiers—as Arthur Frank has called them.[8] That is to say, they serve to bring

7. Bishop, "Rejecting Medical Humanism," 15–25.
8. Frank, "Health Stories as Connectors and Subjectifiers," 421–40.

the sick from patient to agent, from passive to active. In fact, these movements hope to give the patient a kind of power over their disease, a power not accessible to their doctors.

One such movement is the e-patient movement.[9] As Ostherr notes: "The e-patient movement is central to understanding how the voices of patients like Devan Stahl have grown louder in the digital age, because this movement is focused on using digital tools to create access to information and connection to geographically dispersed communities, for the purpose of meeting healthcare needs."[10] The point is that patients are given power over their information, and presumably some sort of power over their bodies, simply because they can now know what the doctor knows. Somehow they take power from the doctor's "objective" view in being given their own "data." "In this way, the whole idea of the e-patient movement is disruptive, because it challenges long-held orthodoxies and power structures in medicine."[11]

By taking over the data, and by giving it to her sister, Devan seems to be attempting to take some sort of ownership over her body, having wrested it away from the doctors. Or at least that seems to be Ostherr's interpretation.

> Goldin Stahl did not adapt the imaging studies simply because they were aesthetically interesting source material, though they certainly have served that function. Instead, she adapted the original clinical images because they had positioned Devan as an object of medical investigation, without agency, voice, or power to resist. Darian's adaptation of those images offers a new interpretation that restores some of the power of self-presentation to the figure in the image, while also exploring the instability often felt by those occupying the subjective role of the "patient."[12]

9. Ferguson, "e-patients: How They Can Help Us Heal Healthcare."

10. Ostherr, "TechnoVision," 63, in this volume.

11. Ibid.

12. Ibid., 66.

There is of course something to what Ostherr is saying here. Subjects who are often subjected to the power of medicine are turned into objects, objects to be manipulated by those in the powerful subject position. That is Foucault's point about the power of the gaze. Yet, if Ostherr is correct, the artist sees Devan's body as a mere object to be manipulated, and thus without agency, voice, or power. If Ostherr is correct, Devan's body, or at least her images, become mere material for the creation of art. In this way of thinking about art, the artist only shifts the node of agential power to a different subject-function. Does the artist not treat Devan's body as an object? If this were the whole story, would the artist not also be complicit in the power ontology that animates much of the Western imaginary? Wouldn't the artist, like the doctor, not also think of her materials as mere objects that function to gain some sort of interpretative control? Wouldn't the artist say to Devan, here is a new way to assert control or ownership over your body? Wouldn't the artist be complicit in the same power ontology, and say that even though the power in the body's functioning is being lost, here is a new kind of psychological power to assert over the body? If we accept the power ontology at work, not only in modern medicine, but also in the entire social imaginary of the late-modern West, then it would seem the only moves left are power moves to wrest power from the powerful doctors—and other powerful structures—and to put it back in the hands of patients. Yet, it seems to me this is not what Darian Stahl is doing, a point to which I shall turn momentarily.

Likewise, drawing on the work of Arthur Frank, Therese Jones points to the way in which patients' narratives tend to follow a typology: a typology that permits the storyteller (or the listener) to engage in a process "constructing and reconstructing" illness stories and identities.[13] The restitution narrative is a story where illness is rendered as "transitory and fix-able."[14] Chaos narratives, on the other hand, are just that. It is almost as if the person is going

13. Jones, "'The becoming of my life. . . ,'" 50, in this volume; Frank, *The Wounded Storyteller*, 1995: 75–96.

14. Ibid., 51; Frank, *The Wounded Storyteller*, 97–114.

to succumb to the chaos of her life; "contingency and uncertainty" will overpower her. These are the hallmarks of chaos narratives.[15] Quest narratives are the third type, which find the protagonist moving from one understanding to another; characteristic of this type of narrative is "automythology, the rebirth or reinvention of the self."[16] Notice that these forms of narrative each serve as a way to overpower the disease, but in a different way than the doctor overpowers the disease. The narratives *psychologically* overpower the disease. Even in the chaos narrative in which there is no resolution, there is a sense in which the narrative itself brings about some sort of control over the chaos. A certain narrative distance gives one a kind of psychological control over the illness.

I certainly see elements of what Ostherr and Jones write about in this volume, namely the self-creating/or self-recreating dimension of the work done by Devan and Darian. Yet, it seems that Ostherr and Jones have accepted the power ontology that animates so much of the West, including much of the work of one of my favorite philosophers, Michel Foucault. One simply has to overcome the entropy at work in the body, if not by the power of medical technology, then by the power of self-creating, self-narrating, by the power of owning one's own agency, becoming the sovereign over the meaning of one's own life.

Yet, it seems to me that this is just a form of self-control, of the empirico-transcendental doublet, of the sovereign-subject, of the solipsistic self. It is a form of self-idolatry, as Marion means it. It is a form of idolatry, doomed to collapse in on itself. The sovereign self gazes upon the subject self, constituting itself in itself and for itself, collapsing the self in on itself. We see here, not the unbearable lightness of being, but the unbearable heaviness of self-constitution, which, it seems to me, collapses in on itself. This image is not a life-giving icon, but a self-destructive idol.

---

15. Jones, "'The becoming of my life. . .,'" 51.

16. Ibid., 11. See Frank, *The Wounded Storyteller*, 115–36.

ICONS OF THE BODY

When flesh comes to mind, and it will always and inevitably come to mind, it is jarring and disruptive of one's self-conception. Flesh calls the self into question. When I look into the mirror and see my gray beard, and the graying hair, I must drop the self-conception that I am still twenty-five years old. How much I have wanted to hide from that reminder of my mortality. The old self is passing away; a new self must come into being, lest I continue to pretend that I am young and become ridiculous to others and myself. I can become self-obsessed if I continually try to remake myself into the twenty-five-year-old.

Let me give an example of what I mean. I trained in medicine in early 1990s, when HIV/AIDS was at its height of its rampage. I can remember several nights running in which every third or fourth admission to the hospital was HIV/AIDS-related; and to make matters worse, about half of those were being admitted to die. I noticed something at that time. If the patient was surrounded by friends and family, if they had others there to occupy their minds, they required less pain medication. And if they were alone or alienated from their friends and family, alone with their own thoughts, they seemed to have more pain, more depression, and more anxiety. While this is certainly only anecdotal, I wonder if it does not name a more general truth. The body seems best suited to stand in the background; it is best suited as a transcendental condition for the possibility of perception and the possibility of agency. In other words, when the body and the self are not objects of the mind, when the body and the self are focused on others, or aimed at projects and purposes, one is most at home in the body. When the flesh is not at the forefront of the mind, one is most at home, most in comfort. We might say that we are at home in our bodies when we are engaged with the world, with others, when we are working toward some purpose. Thus, others call us outside of ourselves and that is when we are given our being.

When her feet and legs started to tingle, the fun stopped. How very badly did Devan want the fun to continue! The hardest part for Devan, at least in her own telling, was the part where she needed to ask for help from Vanderbilt Divinity School. When she needed to ask others into her life, others that might shoulder the burden for her, she could become herself. At first, she could not find the words; but it was the hard work of finding the words in conversation with the school's officials that she finally permitted herself to find the words that appeared in this volume. If she had not sought out others, would she have ever found the words; would this volume even be a possibility? Even that ass-hole of a neurologist (and as a physician I get to call him that) knew that Devan needed something other than his diagnostic skill when he pushed the tissues over to her. And experiencing the neurologist push those tissues over to her—as cold and unfeeling as it was—Devan knew that she herself needed more than the tissues and more than the diagnosis. She needed the assistance of another.

By her own admission, Devan knew that she did not like to cry in front of others; she admits that she likes being in control of herself. And she admits that in her family, there is a way in which sharing those images of her own body, she opens a space for her sister and the rest of her family to speak. In these images she is stripped of clothes, and her own interior—her own bones, her own intestines, her own uterus, her own breasts—are on display; and in not turning inward, in being open to others, she opens a space for her sister to occupy her mind. Devan shares all of those images with her sister, Darian. And in sharing those images, Darian is transformed and Devan is transformed; and together they are now able to talk about her illness. These images act in the way that icons act. They act if we let their power wash over us, if we let the vulnerability of the being whose image it is challenge our preconceptions about ourselves, interrupting our gazes. These images interrupt even Devan's own self-gaze.

And Darian, artist that she is, knows that she must do something with these images. But what? She does not know, at first. She even has to invent new techniques, and explore new materials, in order to enable Devan's MRI images to speak to us. Darian cannot merely manipulate the images, she must press her own hips, her own breasts, her own face, even her entire body over the images. She wraps those cold and revealing images of Devan's body in her own body, giving them warmth and new life. Darian's own flesh is given in these icons and given to Devan, who can now receive them, permitting her normally self-controlling tendency to be overcome by the beauty of what was once a monster. Devan can now receive her own frailty, the gift of her own image, wrapped in the warmth and love of Darian's body. Devan did not assert control over her own body, she surrendered her images to her sister. Darian did not simply hand Devan a manipulated image, she gave her own creative energies and her own body to transform the image into an icon.

One such icon hangs on my wall. A gift has been given to me; it still calls to me every morning from my wall. It calls me out of myself. It calls me to the beauty possible in the darker gifts of the flesh, and calls me to reach out to all the other Devan's in the world. After all, the darker gifts of the flesh eventually come to mind for all of us. It calls me to permit the power of those darker gifts of the flesh to challenge me to respond with the artist's touch, to lovingly make something new for someone else. And in making something new for another, whose flesh fails them, I might just be given my own being.

And in giving us this book, Devan and Darian permit this icon of the body to challenge its readers to reconsider their own experiences with the darker gifts of the flesh, passing the gift along, regiving them again and again, in a non-identical way. In giving us their commentary, Kirsten and Therese expose themselves to my critical philosophical gaze, where I have tried to overpower them with Foucault. When in truth, if I let them be, in my heart of hearts, I know that they do not intend to recapitulate the power ontology regnant within contemporary medicine. I know they too have been touched by these icons of the body, the darker gifts of Devan's flesh, transformed by the love of Darian's artistic hand. And in asking me to comment for this volume, Devan once again gives me a gift, this gift that calls me to set aside my doctor's gaze and my philosopher's gaze, which I wield too easily like a scalpel cutting flesh. In giving us these icons of the body, in giving herself to us in this way, we are made new by these icons. And Devan is made new in giving them. And in giving me this opportunity to comment, to set aside my various gazes, Devan makes me a changed man, a richer man, a new creation. She gives new purpose to my own being.

BIBLIOGRAPHY

Bishop, Jeffrey P. *The Anticipatory Corpse: Medicine, Power, and the Care of the Dying*. Notre Dame, IN: University of Notre Dame Press, 2011.

———. "From Anticipatory Corpse to Posthuman God." *Journal of Medicine and Philosophy* 41 (2016) 679–95.

———. "Rejecting Medical Humanism." *Journal of Medical Humanities* 29 (2008) 15–25.

———. "Transhumanism, Metaphysics, and the Posthuman God." *Journal of Medicine and Philosophy* 35 (2010) 700–720.

Carel, Havi. *Illness: The Cry of the Flesh*. New York: Routledge, 2014.

Cassell, Eric. *The Nature of Suffering and the Goals of Medicine*. 2nd ed. New York: Oxford University Press, 2004.

Ferguson, Tom, with the e-Patients Scholars Working Group. "e-patients: How They Can Help Us Heal Healthcare" (2007). http://e-patients.net.

Foucault, Michel. *The Birth of the Clinic: An Archeology of Medical Perception*. New York: Pantheon, 1994.

———. *The Hermeneutics of the Subject: Lectures at the Collee De France 1981–1982*. Edited by Francois Ewald and Alessandro Fontanta. Translated by Graham Burchell. New York: Picador, 2001.

Frank, Arthur. "Health Stories as Connectors and Subjectifiers." *Health: An Interdisciplinary Journal for the Social Study of Health, Illness and Medicine* 10 (2006) 421–40.

———. *The Wounded Storyteller: Body, Illness, and Ethics*. Chicago: University of Chicago Press, 1995.

Heidegger, Martin. *Being and Time*. Translated by Joan Stambaugh. Albany, NY: State University of New York Press, 2010.

Marion, Jean-Luc. *God Without Being*. Translated by Thomas A. Carlson. Chicago: University of Chicago Press, 1991.

Toombs, S. Kay. *The Meaning of Illness: A Phenomenological Account of the Different Perspectives of Physician and Patient*. New York: Springer, 1992.

for the overall project, but these authors subvert the particularity of my story. By placing my narrative within the more general discourses of their disciplinary fields, the authors of this volume help to universalize my experience. Darian expresses the paradox between the particular and universal explicitly in chapter 2. The lived experience of impairment is always particular, but its effects are widespread. Not only does the impairment of one member of our society affect many other members, but most people, if they live long enough, will eventually find themselves impaired. Compelling narratives are always about a particular person or event, but what makes them impactful is their ability to resonate with a wide variety of people. The same is true of fine art. When attending gallery openings with Darian, our hope is not that people will learn something about me, but that they will learn something about what it is like to live with chronic illness that resonates with their own experience. Viewing Darian's art, therefore, should engender empathy. This volume is an extension of the mission of our initial collaboration. I will not endeavor to respond to each chapter of this volume individually, though each chapter is rich enough for a direct response; instead, I will reflect upon themes that arose between the works that I found particularly illuminating or challenging. I begin with the tension that arose in many chapters concerning resistance, power, and submission. Many have interpreted my narrative and my collaboration with Darian as a form of resistance against biomedicine, which empowers patients such as myself. I grant that empowerment is a product of this resistance, but in my case, empowerment comes through submission—I choose to submit my body to medicine, but I also submit my narrative and medical images to the authors and readers of this volume. Next, I reflect on the theme of identity-formation that arose in many of the chapters. Several of the authors positioned my narrative into larger narrative schemes and positioned me as a member of growing resistance and liberation movements. Given my emerging membership into such groups, I reflect upon the theme of intersectionality and multiplicity, which arose in some of the chapters. Finally, I consider the theme of transformation. Many of the authors of this volume pressed me to consider how I understand the purpose of my body and the purpose of this project. Becoming broken, fragmented, and liminal is ontologically transformative, as is learning to see yourself through another's lens.

RESISTANCE, POWER, AND SUBMISSION

One of the clearest themes throughout these chapters is the idea of resistance. Most people first come to learn of their chronic illness in the medical system, and it is tempting to allow the biomedical model of disease to control our thinking about chronic illness. The authors of this volume, however, believe the medical system is limited in its ability to understand and care for ill patients. This is not to say the authors begrudge or revile medicine; rather, they appreciate that medicine is a cultural product with a bounded scope. Bishop in particular notes how medicine has separated the purpose of the body from its function, so that clinicians can focus on returning the body to normal functioning. If my physician were as concerned with the purpose of my body, or my self-conception, as my body's function, it might distract him from his goal of restoring the functioning of my body.[1] The bounded scope of the physician's job is not a problem necessarily—my physician ought not to endeavor to be my friend, counselor, or chaplain. The problem comes when the physician's singular understanding of the body prevents him from expressing empathy for his patients, or when his reliance upon the medical image becomes an idol that prevents him from seeing his patient's humanity. All people are multidimensional, and when we reduce a person to a single representation, we make idols of their image.

Similarly, Armour describes the tendency of biomedicine to reduce ill people to objects in the service of biopower. Biopower reflects our ways of knowing, and biomedicine harnesses biopower to construct "what is known, how it's known, and who knows it."[2]

1. Bishop, "Icons of the Body, Darker Gifts of the Flesh," 97, in this volume.

2. Armour, "Artful Self-Reflection as Biomedical Intervention," 78, in this volume.

Within biomedicine, my body is known through a particular set of visual techniques that see the body in a particular way. The techno-visual medical gaze, enabled in part by advanced medical imaging machines, such as MRI machines, comes to be the primary way physicians *see* some illnesses. In turn, medical images can become the primary way physicians see their patients. The MRI machine produces images that are understood as true representations. Ostherr notes medical visualizations require interpretation, but also halt interpretation. They help provide a diagnosis where there once was only a hypothesis.[3] The surety by which my physician diagnosed me after seeing my MR images testifies to the power of medical imaging in medicine. Of course, as Ostherr explains, these imagining technologies are part of a complex network of meaning production.[4] Although MR images have an important function in medicine, their meaning is not self-evident, nor should it be taken for granted. Darian and I, along with the authors in this volume, are attempting to resist the singular medical interpretation of MR images.

Resistance, of course, does not mean shunning or triumphing over medicine. I choose to be involved in the medical system. As Jones points out, my narrative expresses the tension of being both willing and forced to participate in medicine. I willingly subject myself to the power of medicine, but I do so reluctantly, subtly resisting the ways in which it reduces me. I resist biomedical subjection,[5] even while participating in the biomedical system as a research subject, patient, and now as a clinical ethicist. Participating in the medical system allows me to access the goods of medicine, such as drug therapies, symptom management, and high-tech monitoring of the progression of my disease. I am grateful to be able to access these medical goods and I am reticent to criticize our healthcare system in a time in which so many Americans lack necessary access to it. There is much in medicine worth

3. Ostherr, "TechnoVision," 58, in this volume.
4. Ibid.
5. Armour, "Artful Self-Reflection as Biomedical Intervention," 82.

supporting, but it is an imperfect system that requires reform and resistance.

Resistance can be difficult, but it can also be empowering. Engaging the medical system as a patient can be a disempowering experience. As I described in my narrative, to access the goods of medicine, I must submit my body to others and rely on the knowledge and expertise of physicians. The plan to give my medical images to Darian, however, was not initially conceived as a way to take ownership over my image or as an act of empowerment. The images were for Darian, not for myself. Possessing and perusing them without my physician present, however, was empowering. It was really the act of Darian's creativity, however, that felt most empowering. I had submitted my images once more to a professional, but through submission, I was able to gain some ownership of my image. The difference between Darian and my physician is that Darian sees me as a collaborator and not as an object to be investigated.

As Ostherr and Armour note, resistance requires creativity and vulnerability. Both were necessary for my collaboration with Darian and the goals of our project. Because I do not wish to escape the medical system, we must imagine more subtle ways to avoid the medical model of disease. My and Darian's collaboration resists the biomedical way of seeing and knowing the body. After presenting reflections on our collaboration at a bioethics conference, I was asked why I do not create my own art. Would it not be more empowering and satisfying if I had full ownership over my body's representation? Would it not be more healing or more therapeutic to create the art myself? Beyond the fact that I could never hope to replicate my sister's awesome talent, there is something to be gained in giving over the power of my body's image to another. The inability to own your image can be oppressive, but giving that image away can also be liberating. Because I do not create the art, I have critical distance from it. Allowing another person to reshape my body allows me to see the images as universal—they exceed me and invite others to see themselves reflected in her art.

Likewise, the authors of this volume work to resist what Armour terms the "theo-logic" of biomedicine by calling attention to it and offering alternative understandings of the ill body and its place in academic discourse, social structures, and our cultural imagination. For this to happen, however, I first had to admit my own vulnerability. I had to acknowledge that I needed others to help me resist the biomedical gaze and I needed to hand over my story and images to others to allow them to collaborate with me in resistance. Silence is typical after a person becomes ill, because, as Jones notes, chronic illness is alienating and confusing.[6] Silence in the face of illness is protective. Armour observes that Darian's piece, "Numb," reflects the self-protection I first sought after I was diagnosed. It is not surprising, therefore, that this was the first image Darian made about me. She did not yet have access to my MR images and my silence on the topic was aptly expressed as cold self-preservation. Reading Darian's chapter, I was struck by how our familial silence affected each of us. Wrapped up in my own struggles, I had not considered how my diagnosis would affect those close to me, including my family. Breaking my silence was generative and enabled the art Darian has presented. All this to say, there can be power in submission. As Bishop describes, surrendering my images to Darian allowed me to receive my image anew. Giving Darian the gift of my broken body, she was able to give it back to me—more whole and intact than I had presented it to her. Together we helped to create an icon, rather than an idol.

IDENTITY FORMATION

I believe the composition of this volume reflects how many people experience illness. Illness, particularly chronic illness, cannot be confined to a single sphere of one's life. Rather, illness permeates multiple parts of a person's life and creates multiple identities. The image we have of ourselves is never determined by us alone; instead, it is constructed, or rather *co*-constructed, in our

6. Jones, "The becoming of my life . . . ," 46, in this volume.

interactions with other individuals and through our environment. In addition to medical professionals, others help to inform how I understand my illness-identity: my family members, fellow MS patients, professional colleagues, my environment, and the complex social systems in which I reside. My self-image, or body image, therefore, is not singular. The phenomenologist Gail Weiss, whose writing helped to inspire this volume, explains,

> Images of the body are not discrete but form a series of overlapping identities whereby one or more aspects of that body appear to be especially salient at any given point in time. . . . [B]ody images . . . are copresent in any given individual, and . . . are themselves constructed through a series of corporeal exchanges that take place both within and outside of specific bodies.[7]

In each chapter of this volume, I see myself through a new lens and a new body image predominates my imagination. Some of these images are familiar, but others are challenging. Various authors describe me, and others like me, in ways that I struggle to reconcile with my self-understanding. This not to say I feel compelled to take up or incorporate these multiple versions of myself into my body image; rather, the chapters challenge me to see myself through the eyes of another.

Darian's art challenges me to consider my identity outside of medicine. Even though I resist medicine's reductionist tendencies, my narratives about MS are largely situated in the clinic. It is difficult for me to break away from associating my illness with medical spaces. Darian's art, however, places my body in more domestic spaces. Darian, of course, does not know me as a patient. She has never accompanied me to a doctor's visit. Darian knows me in domestic spaces that we have inhabited together. Darian knows that I do not leave my MS behind when I get home. When she imagines my ill body, it carries the MR images around in the background of my daily life. Her image of me as a domestic dweller is equally as accurate as my narrative portrayal of myself as a medical patient.

7. Weiss, *Body Images*, 2.

Darian's images are more salient in the spaces I inhabit most often. As often as I go to my doctor's office, I spend much more time at home, wondering about my illness, wondering whether I tripped because of MS, dropped my keys because of MS, or am tired because of MS. Darian's art brings to the fore the persisting questions that rest in the background of my consciousness. Why do I rarely write about these moments? Perhaps because these moments are more intimate and more personal. Darian based her prints on stories I told about my life with MS, but I tell many stories, and most are not about my home life. Yet, this is where Darian focuses—this is the part of my identity she foregrounds. Her domestic focus adds another dimension to my body image.

Other authors of this volume shed light on the parts of my identity that I downplay. Before this volume, I considered my resistance to biomedicine to be subtly subversive. I am not the MS warrior I hear described in other narratives and I did not necessarily consider myself part of a group of activists or part of a social justice movement. The authors of this volume portray me as much more courageous and more of an activist than I typically see myself. Upon reflection, however, resistance and activism can take on many forms, and narrative and art have a long history of subversive protest.

Ostherr also reminds me that I belong to groups that I do not acknowledge, even if they understand my work as part of their mission. I was unfamiliar with the e-patient movement before reading Ostherr's chapter. My resistance to particular medical practices predominantly takes place outside of the clinic, although I appreciate movements that encourage patients to participate in their medical care. Ostherr helped to remind me that the ease with which I was able to obtain a copy of my MRI scans is likely the product of people like "e-patient Dave" who helped to ensure patients had access their medical records.[8] Likewise, I benefit from the HIV/AIDS activists who struggled to control their public representations. I was under no illusion that Darian and I were doing something radically new in our collaboration, but I failed

8. Ostherr, "TechnoVision," 65.

to acknowledge the disease activists who laid the foundation for our project. Unlike those early activists, I do not struggle to find information about my disease or lack access to medical research or disease-modifying therapies, but I continue the fight to control my image. I am a part of a second wave of activists who use their medical access and knowledge to resist certain aspects of the medical culture. Acknowledging my place within these larger patient movements inspires me to see myself as an activist. Belonging to activist groups also encourages me to consider my ethical obligations to other patients like myself and to patient activist movements more generally. This new image of myself morally binds me to others.

Not only am I bound to patient groups because of my illness, my embodiment also places me into other social categories I do not always acknowledge. As Armour points out, I am not only chronically ill and female; I am also white, straight, cis-gendered, middle class, and educated. As a woman, I am keenly aware of instances in which my gender shapes my encounters with medical professionals, some of which I described in my narrative. In other ways, however, my multiple (and intersecting) identities privilege me in medical spaces. My resistance to aspects of the medical system I find oppressive rests on my ability to access the medical system in the first place. I benefit from a job that provides me with health insurance and allows me access to multiple physicians and expensive medications. Once inside the clinic, I do not struggle with the way the medical model defines my gender and sexuality, the size and shape of my body, or clinicians' racial bias and other kinds of bias patients face when encountering medical professionals. I also benefit from being taken seriously in the domains I occupy. My credentials now afford me a certain respect from physicians I had not previously experienced. Acknowledging my privilege allows me to imagine the ways in which I relate to other patients, and reminds me that my experience will not resonate with many other MS patients who will need space to tell their own stories.

TRANSFORMATION

Because this volume challenges my self-understanding and adds additional meaning to my illness identity, it has a transformative power. Being diagnosed as chronically ill has its own transformative power. As Bishop attests, it is easy to take one's body for granted when all is well. Flesh becomes noticeable, or present at hand, when it fails.[9] I experienced my body this way during my first MS relapse, when my feet and legs became numb. I continue to experience this when my body prevents me from doing what I intended to do, such as climbing the stairs or reading my computer screen. The unity with which I experience myself in the world ruptures in these moments. My illness not only subverts my desires in the spaces I presently occupy, but it also changes the way I understand my temporal existence. During relapse, it is difficult to think about the future because the difficulty of functioning demands a preoccupation with the present. When in remission, on the other hand, it is easy to project all present functioning into the future. A physical or mental slip up can be a sign of a symptom to come. Even when my body is functioning normally, I am often aware that such instances of bodily coherence might be fleeting.

Chronic illness, therefore, is a part of my identity, because it has transformed how I experience and interact with the world. Jones is correct in identifying my experience as prolonged liminality. Looking well while being ill places me in a liminal category, somewhere between healthy and sick. I am in the process of becoming something new, of being transformed as Victor Turner might say.[10] I can only hope my refashioning is endowing me with new powers to cope going forward.[11] Even when the time comes when I look ill or disabled, I will remain liminal in other respects. MS will continue to cause interruptions in my life. I imagine my future narrative will likely continue to have elements of chaos because of the relapsing remitting nature of my disease. I will be

9. Bishop, "Icons of the Body, Darker Gifts of the Flesh," 96.

10. Turner, *The Forest of Symbols*.

11. Jones, "'The becoming of my life. . . ,'" 46.

charged continuously with adjusting to a new bodily reality. Holding the fragments of my life and identity together in ambiguity has ontological value.[12] I do not simply have new knowledge because of my illness; I also have a new ontology. Knowledge and wisdom, as Jones notes, re-make me.[13]

Darian's art represents and contributes to my refashioning. In her art, Darian gives me back the parts of my body that most clearly represent me to the world. In the MR image, I am anonymous to nearly all who know me. In much of Darian's art, however, I have a face, a body, and a story. Darian's flesh gives her art a body, but we share that flesh through our sisterly bond. Pressing her flesh into my image, Darian gives me a part of herself to incorporate into my image. Sharing flesh, we co-create my image and we are both transformed. As Bishop points out, Darian helps make beauty out of something that was monstrous.[14] Monstrosity sets one apart, makes a person alien and aberrant, according the Latin word *monstrum* from which the word derives. Medieval broadsides and modern books of teratology single out monsters as liminal—human, but also not quite human. Seeing oneself as monstrous is to see oneself as separate from the rest of humanity. Belonging and yet not belonging to the human race. Darian has pieces that represent this feeling of being set apart through monstrosity.

12. Ibid., 40.
13. Ibid.
14. Bishop, "Icons of the Body, Darker Gifts of the Flesh," 05.

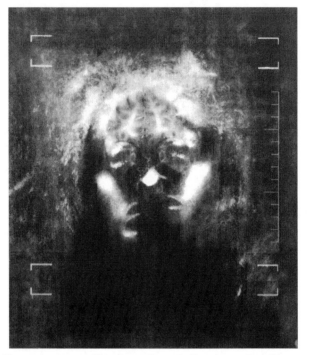

"Becoming Scanned," Lithography and silkscreen, 30" x 28" 2014

Darian does not leave me here, however. She acknowledges the feeling of alienation that can come through being ill, but by being present to me in her art, she ensures that I am not left alone.

Armour hints at, but backs away from the language of transubstantiation to describe what Darian's art is doing. I challenge Darian not to think of her work as merely translation, but as transubstantiation. Darian not only represents my body but also becomes a part of my body. In the act of creating art, my body is transformed. The result is not simply a modified MRI, although the art retains the MR image, the result is a new body. Darian may see her art as representing my embodied narrative, but its impact circles back to me, continually transforming me and demanding new representations, which emerge because of our collaboration. Our ontology, therefore, is participatory, mutually transformed in participation with one another through the act of creation.

CONCLUSION

Pathographies of triumph over disease abound. Readers enjoy stories where disease sufferers ultimately win. The classic tale of good triumphing over evil is reinscribed in these stories and assures the public that fragile creatures can win their battle with the evils of mortality. Quest journeys, stories of living with illness and learning from illness, are less dramatic and less death-defying. MS is not my enemy, however; it is, as Bishop names it, my darker gift of the flesh. MS shapes the way my body functions and interacts with my world. It transforms how I relate to others. It has placed itself at the core of my embodied becoming. This is how most people will experience their bodies as they age—not as triumph, but as reluctant acceptance of our fragility. Resilience is necessary, but there are few models for it. I hope this volume will encourage others who are chronically ill or impaired, to write themselves into wellbeing and allow others to share in the process of mutual transformation through resistant acts of creation.

BIBLIOGRAPHY

Turner Victor. *The Forest of Symbols: Aspects of Ndembu Ritual.* Ithaca, NY: Cornell University Press, 1967.

Weiss, Gail. *Body Images: Embodiment as Intercorporeality.* New York: Routledge, 1999.